Praise for the knowledge Hannah Pilnick reveals in her books and seminars:

"*I wish for everyone to be exposed to this work. Peace will prevail not only in our lives and the lives of our children, but in the whole world.*"

—*MIRI GOLDIN, Ph.D., Neuroscientist Researcher*

"As *an opera singer I have a very stressful life and must stay in great shape physically, mentally, and vocally. I have used this knowledge many times to prevent getting sick during rehearsals and needing to take antibiotics. It has also made it possible for me to open up more and more and become the artist I have dreamed of becoming.*

Hannah gave me tools to face my deepest fears and to heal myself."

—*ALMA SADE, World Renowned Opera Singer*

"*For fifteen years my life was ruled by migraines. I took 15 pills a month. I used to go around at home bitter and pessimistic. I did not feel I took part in the joy of life— until I first met with the Healing Parents knowledge.*

After many years of terrible suffering, I have healed myself. Now, if I have an occasional migraine, I am reminded that cleansing work lasts a lifetime. I am not the same woman whose life was ruled by migraines anymore; today I am directed by my deepest inner self."

—*RINA RAVE, Senior Instructor of Rehabilitative Art*

"After three long, painful years in which I went through 18 in vitro fertilizations (IVFs), I came to Hannah who showed me the light in the terrible darkness. She taught me how to light my life and my womb. Two months later I became pregnant and today I am a happy mother to three enlightened children."

—LITAL OHEV ZION

"We felt so helpless when we got the news from the doctors that our newborn daughter was very sick and that her life was in danger. The baby was anesthetized, hooked up to a respirator, and connected to so many tubes—a very hard scene to watch. We couldn't even touch her. But the healing powers that exist within us mothers, and about which I have learned from Hannah's Healing Parents knowledge, led to the longed-for change. We succeeded, Hannah and I, to treat my little baby using Hannah's CCH techniques. Just one week after her birth, my daughter was released from the intensive care unit. The doctors were astonished. They did not believe it possible that our child could recover from her condition at all, and certainly not so quickly.

Thank you, Hannah, for teaching me about the immense powers latent within me and my abilities to treat my loved ones."

—OSHRA AICORT

"There is no greater pain in the world than that of a mother whose child suffers and whom she cannot help in any way.

When my son was first diagnosed with sever autism, with cognitive and speech delays, I felt the world was painted black. Pain and sorrow penetrated every organ in my body and into my soul. I felt helpless and frightened.

Miraculously, I came to hear a lecture given by Hannah and she immediately embraced me with endless warmth and love. The wisdom and accessibility of the Healing Parents knowledge gave me the security and the power to heal my son. Thanks to this knowledge I know that from now on our way is lit and the darkness in our lives is now replaced with a vibrant and colorful world.

My son's condition improved immediately, and within one and a half years of intensive work with the Healing Parents knowledge and tools, it was determined by experts that he was no longer autistic. In fact, he tested above average in cognitive abilities for his age.

Hannah taught me the power of love, and how a mother's love to her son can change the world. Always.

For that I will be eternally grateful."

—DANA WEINBERG

"*Before attending Hannah's workshop, for several years my marriage life was going downhill. I was angry at life, miserable, desperate, hurt and was blaming my husband for making my life such a pain. My kids were sick from time to time and were very confused about their lives. I had one foot out the door in my marriage.*

When I started the workshop, I saw myself changing. Then a miracle that I didn't expect happened: my family changed. I understood it was I who was the cause; my family was a reflection of me.

Since then my marriage life improved day by day. My kids got happier & healthier. I became a loving mother, wife, and a better person.

Hannah gave me a simply healthy & joyful life as a gift."

—*DORIT DE LUCA*

"I was in great pain, and fear controlled my life. I also lived with immense frustration from all the traumas I went through. Inside I felt angry and bitter, but I was always pleasing others and repressed my own feelings. Today, I see everything in a different light. I went through a long journey of healing. I have eliminated frustrations, fears, and many angers from my life. The knowledge helped me heal my body and my soul.

This book gave me deep insights in every aspect of my life and I understood that everything is in our hands and that we can change our lives and heal our body and spirit in the cleansing process.

Now I take greater responsibility for my life. Every day I observe myself and check what I can improve. It has become an integral part of my life. I use it to heal myself and my grandchildren. Every day I wake up in the morning and the knowledge is with me.

I give thanks to the Creator of this world that brought me a child that lit my life.

And to you my most beloved daughter, thank you for enlightening my heart."

—LILI LEVY, *Mother to Hannah Pilnick*

the Gift

THE POWER
OF PARENTING

" Your children are an external picture of your deepest inner self. They reflect what has been hidden, repressed & concealed for years. They cry out your inner pain—through mental, emotional, and physical suffering—so that you are able to see it and remove it from your life.

They are your most loyal bodyguards.

They will guard you in every way, even at the price of taking your suffering upon themselves and risking their own lives. "

— Hannah Pilnick

Prologue

My first encounters with the awareness that I affect the life of my son felt more like a burden than a gift. It all started a few weeks after my son's birth. However, it took nearly a year for this realization to crystallize.

The moment in which I started to clearly understand my affect on him remains forever imprinted in my heart. It was then that I saw that who I am on the inside directly affects who he is and who he will grow up to be. I remember that morning so clearly. My son was screaming at home and I was looking at him, understanding that he was crying my distress and my pain. In that moment, all my experience as a therapist aligned. I became one with the universe, connected with all, yet the world around me stood frozen. There was only my son and me. I saw my suffering through him and heard the beats of fear in my heart as I grasped how my pain was causing his suffering.

Here I am doing everything I can in order to be a good mother, and suddenly it all explodes in my face. In this one moment, through this one-year-old baby standing helpless before me, I can see myself clearly. I watch his suffering and know that it is because of me.

Burning tears flowed from my eyes, and a deep sadness surrounded me. I was frozen with fear. But then my child approached me and hugged me, and everything shifted. The warmth of his body, his kind, loving eyes, and my immense love towards him, melted me and brought me immediately back to reality. I breathed him into myself, and within seconds the beats of fear turned to beats of joy. A wave of love and hope flowed through me.

From a nightmare of guilt and fear a gift was born; the biggest gift I could ask for. I embraced my son and enveloped him with my love. I knew I was not the same mother anymore; I was not the same person anymore. At that moment, I embarked on a new life journey with one clear goal: maintaining my son's emotional and physical health. I became determined to apply anything and everything in order to achieve this goal.

I chose to begin a cleansing journey that will last for the rest of my life; a journey in which I do not blame, but observe myself and take full responsibility for my actions, thoughts, and intentions. I understood that I am the creator of my life and that I influence the life of my child and the generations to come. I understood that by focusing on my cleansing, I could maintain my health and prevent much suffering from my child.

True, it is not easy to persist in a cleansing journey, but it is much harder to see and to cope with a suffering child.

I was faced with the truth that day, and chose to take it into my life. That same day, I planted a seed in my heart, that I would do everything possible to unite parents to work together towards one clear goal: to prevent suffering and uproot it from the lives of children. The seed has developed and with the years turned into a beautiful tree that bears fruit. These fruits shared within this book are my gift to you.

the Gift

The Power Of Parenting

Hannah Pilnick

www.healingparents.net

The Gift
THE POWER OF PARENTING

Hannah Pilnick

Heavens
Publishing

info@heavenspublishing.com

BCAF

Acknowledgements

My dear Mother, Lili, the one and only: Thank you for all your devotion and for your unconditional love. Thank you for all your help and acceptance, and for enabling me to be who I am.

Nadav, my dear husband: Thank you for all your love, devotion, and loyalty to me and to our children. Thank you for your tireless dedication, giving your daily support and hard work unconditionally to help make my life mission come true.

My Dear Children, Jonathan, Naama, and David: Each one of you, in your unique way, has opened my heart and has pushed me to be a better person. My sweet, beloved dears, thank you for showing consideration and support at such a young age.

Liat, my long-time friend: Thank you for being there for me along the way.

Orit, my dear friend: Thank you for your benevolence and devotion to my family and to our vision.

Lena and Stephanie: Your editing skills and dedication helped in making this book clearer and more precise.

And finally, *to all my Patients*: Thank you for enabling me to take part in your personal life journey. I learned much from each and every one of you, and today I impart the experience I gained through you to the whole world.

Contents

PART D THE FORMULA

CCH Techniques and Exercises

🔊 An audio CD which guides you through these techniques, *"The Gift: The Power of Parenting | CCH Techniques,"* can be purchased separately at www.healingparents.net or on amazon.com. See "Book and Audio CD Order Information" at the end of this book.

Introduction

Envision a world free from suffering. This is a world in which children do not depend on medication or treatments in order to live, in which there is no disease or life-threatening situations among children, and children are free from physical, mental, and emotional limitations. Envision these children free to fulfill their own dreams.

I work every day to turn this vision, which is our true nature, into a universal way of life.

I hear the cries of mothers and see the hearts of fathers torn by their children's suffering. Though our own children may not be suffering, when we look around us see countless children who are. Every day, I encounter the suffering of people. Most of us feel helpless, not knowing how to ease other's pain, thinking only, "Heaven forbid this should happen to us." *Yet everyone can do something*. All of humanity is inextricably tied. When one child suffers, the whole world suffers. So too, when each of us takes part in helping to ease the pain of our loved ones, the whole world begins to heal. We must end the suffering of all children. You can play a significant role in this shift by starting in your own home.

I am about to reveal to you the *"Healing Parents"* knowledge and enable you to take whatever you need from the knowledge for yourself and your loved ones. By using this knowledge, you will get an opportunity to go through a personal cleansing process, which will maintain your health and the health of your children. In this way, together, we can help ensure that the next generations will enjoy a life free of suffering.

Does this seem unrealistic? I am telling you, it is *already happening*. The shift has begun, and if each one of you takes part in this mission, in a few years we will see the world change. For this mission, my work alone is not enough. For this mission I need everyone.

This generation, our generation, must make great strides for the sake of future generations. We have to join in and take action now.

And as to you, dear children, I promise you that I will dedicate my entire life for the sake of this goal and will pass on any information I possess to the world, while cleansing myself in every way possible. Thus, you and the generations that follow will get to enjoy a healthy life, full of satisfaction and love, living in peace with yourselves, with each other, with the universe, and with the Creator.

I love you and give you this book with great love and devotion.

Hannah

Part A

~

Where Did We Come From And Where Are We Going?

Chapter 1

The Beginning of a Life Journey

We live our lives, perform our everyday obligations, go to work, and manage our family routine. Yet at times, questions emerge: why are we even here and why are things happening to us? Why do our children suffer? Is there something else at play here, something that determines the pace of our lives? What is the formula, the code that leads some of us to live a life replete with goodness while others end up facing frustrations and a life filled with suffering?

Throughout my life, I have asked myself these questions time and again. After a journey of discovery over many years, through intense work with patients having various suffering situations, and through deep inner work, the picture became clear. For me, it was a breakthrough in understanding our role as parents, our purpose in the world, the source of our suffering, and how to distance ourselves and our children from suffering.

When I understood the power and the potential of what I had discovered, I was determined to share it with all the parents in the world. However, it was clear to me that most parents did not possess the knowledge and experience I had in healing. For the most part, parents do not have the confidence that they are able to heal. For some people the knowledge might even contradict things they have learned throughout their lives. I understood I had to organize and write all that I knew, then simplify it and make it applicable to everyone.

When I sat down to write this knowledge for all parents to utilize, I closed my eyes, and then a fascinating thing happened. A torrent of information started flowing through me. I was amazed at what I received, and passionately wrote every word. I sat day after day for seven months and devotedly wrote everything that came to me, including my insights. I was amazed how completely this knowledge matched all my life experiences and my experience as a therapist. It was like watching a movie where the end, and even the next chapter, is not known; a movie about a different lifetime; about our world and a parallel world, immense and fascinating —a world that until then I had only seen while treating people. Through writing, I was able to transfer in a simple and fluent manner knowledge that took me my lifetime to discover.

The first part of this book, starting at the next chapter, consists of what I call "The Story." It is the essence of the flow of information that I mentioned above. Reading and internalizing this story is crucial for successfully making the knowledge in this book part of your life. You might grasp its immense importance right away or it might come to you as you read further on.

In this book, I will share with you insights and knowledge I was privileged to discover, so that you can use them in your everyday life, for your own sake and the sake of your children. I will present to you the basics of the knowledge. You can use this knowledge regardless of your current practices. The knowledge in this book is suitable for all people, not only parents; it will complement any lifestyle. It is what every person needs to know, understand, do, and be, regardless of his personal path, religion, or beliefs, in order to fulfill himself, prevent suffering, and live a healthy life.

I invite you to join me on a fascinating journey. Along the way, three things are required of you: willpower, practice, and persistence. The rest will naturally unfold.

As you read this book, use a dedicated notebook to perform the exercises and take notes. Do not erase anything, just turn the page and continue. Get it all out, from the inside out, onto the pages.

Our journey starts at a magical place found above us, the "higher worlds."

The "higher worlds" is a dynamic living environment of immense scope. It is populated by creatures on different levels. They have incredible order and mutual respect for each other. Everyone there knows their role and is always willing to offer help.

These creatures have no body, but they do have colors. They work around the clock, and some of them can be at an infinite number of places simultaneously.

These creatures have many roles. They are wonderfully organized, so that each one knows its place and purpose.

They are organized in a pyramid, so that the lowest rank is at the bottom of the pyramid, and as they go up they move up a rank, until they get to the top, where the Commander-in-Chief sits. Each rank has its own color, so that if one of the "soldiers," for any reason, gets confused and goes elsewhere, it is returned to its place in line with its color.

In the higher worlds, each enjoys its role, is satisfied with its condition, and loves to help others. There is everything up there, and everything starts from there. What reaches our world arrives after many years of being created in the higher worlds.

Each time, one of these creatures is selected in the higher worlds as suitable to come down and bring the notion which is then perceived in our world as a discovery.

In the higher worlds, each one of the creatures works on developing itself and the group that is commensurate with its developmental stage; the objective each one of them has is to move up a rank in the pyramid, change its color and location, and by so doing get as close as possible to the Commander-in-Chief.

In addition, they can receive support and love from the group located above them.

Something is interrupting my writing. Someone is pulling at my shoulder. Wait, I want to see what this is all about. I turn back and see the charming creatures. "You have not introduced us to your readers," they say. And again, they are of course right. Dear readers, let's make the introductions; the creatures I've been telling you about are called souls.

Now I am relaxed. You know them by their full name—souls. They are made of light, and as I already noted, they come in different colors, and they live in the higher worlds.

Every day our world and the higher worlds are swept into each other and mix with each other. Let yourself go and open up to a new and spectacular world. There is life around you beyond what your five senses are able to detect. You are accustomed to seeing things according to certain shapes, and therefore your ordinary eyes cannot detect them. Yet I am telling you: they are here around us, they are full of strength and courage, they walk and fly, and are bursting with energy and goodwill to help.

Why do they arrive in our world?

They arrive in our world because we summon them. Someone here in this world called them to come; he called for help, whether consciously or not.

This is a good time to share the following with you: The creatures living in the higher worlds are partly people you know; people who are dear to you and who left our world. Some of them are people who left our world and whom we have heard or read about in the Bible and other ancient books. Some of them are angels, such as Michael, Gabriel, and so on.

They are placed in the pyramid in line with their level of consciousness. The higher their rank, the higher they are positioned and able to be at many places simultaneously, responding to many calls. All of them are found there, all of them live there, and all of them can simultaneously live with us too.

This is also something I am eager to share with you: there is no such thing as "death." We all live simultaneously—the difference has to do with where and how.

There are cosmic forces that balance good and bad, strong and weak, stability and instability. In addition, there are cosmic forces that set the balance between the souls found here in our world and the souls found in the higher worlds.

At any given moment, there are souls that arrive in our world, and souls that depart from our world and ascend to the higher worlds.

Those who return to the higher worlds are souls that have completed their mission in our world, while all those who descend from the higher worlds are souls that join our forces, either for a life journey or for a short time in order to help us.

The souls that come to our world in order to help us are ancient, immense, and possess infinite knowledge. They want an invitation and wait for a voice to summon them. They are happy to offer help anytime and they have abilities in any area you can imagine, and also in many fields that we are still unfamiliar with and cannot imagine.

~~~

You know what? I am telling you about the creatures in the higher worlds and I have even introduced them to you as souls, but I have not shared with you how they were created, who created them, or who they belong to.

I have so much to share with you that it is hard to decide where to start. But I have made a decision. I am no longer keeping anything to myself. I am about to tell you the whole story, from the beginning …

Chapter 2

Awakening the Sparks of Light

In the beginning there was no separation between the higher worlds and our world. Everything was one.

Nothing existed except for an immense ball of light. One day, he[1] started moving with great power, shifting around in circular motions, making spiral movements, until he shattered and divided himself into a countless number of balls of light of different colors. Each light ball contained sparks of light. The number of sparks in the different balls of light was not identical. Some balls of light contained ten sparks, others contained two, and yet others contained thousands.

The bang was so great and powerful that all the new balls of light scattered in all directions. An endless space of light balls of differing colors was created.

To the surprise of the great ball of light, he remained precisely as immense and powerful as he was

---

[1] Please note the word "he" is used throughout the book for simplicity; the ball of light has no gender.

before the great bang. He observed the spectacular view he had created and decided that these sparks of light were his family. From then on, he had countless children and was obligated to them. He was happy with what he had. He understood that he loved them greatly and would love them forever, and therefore he decided to share with them equally his strength, light, and power, irrespective of their sizes, color, or location.

The great bang created new life followed by a period of calm. There was still no movement, only utter silence.

One day, the great ball decided to set in motion the life he created. He wanted to awaken his children, to get to know each one of them, to give them some of his power, potency, and knowledge—just as we wish to share with our children. He knew that as they were created from him, each one of them had a part of him in them, and even if it was only a tiny particle, he must awaken it, as it contained all his best. *He assumed this as his greatest mission: awakening the sparks of light; awakening each one of his children.*

He sent a warm ray of light to each one of the balls of light. The rays penetrated deep into each one of them and spread great warmth. The warmth seeped and prompted motion within them. The sparks of light within the balls felt the warmth penetrating them and started to rise. They began to shift within the ball of light in which they were created and started to grasp that they existed. They looked around themselves, and what they saw was life within the ball.

In all the balls, the same thing occurred simultaneously. The sparks within them started to spin around, move in spirals, and fly just like their father, the great ball of light, had done before he shattered.

The great ball observed this and was overjoyed. "They're awake, they're alive," he told himself. He thought that it would be worthwhile to grant the sparks of light a little more time to be with themselves and adjust to the new situation. And so it was that he gave them the time they needed. Inside their respective balls, the sparks of light spun around, got to know each other, and felt each other's presence. They recognized the fact that they were of equal size, color, and shape. They enjoyed the equality and lived in peace. They did not know there were other balls outside their own, nor did they know how they were created. They simply existed.

Time passed, and the great ball sent a second ray of light to each one of the balls of light. Along with this ray of light, he exhaled a strong gust of wind that hit each one of them. This shot of air prompted a powerful motion within the balls and created a sense of unpleasantness. The sparks were used to the warm and relaxed feeling yet suddenly something undermined their tranquil lives. In each ball, the sparks of light converged in the center into one unit and became so still they seemed to be frozen.

The great ball decided to undertake another experiment and sent a warm ray of light into the balls of light. The sparks of light felt the warmth coming in and let go of each other. They went back to a tranquil and comfortable life. Each spark was on its own, flying in spirals and circles within its ball of light. Yet suddenly, the great ball again exhaled a strong gust of wind. The sparks once again converged at the center into one unit, yet were less frightened than the first time. At this stage, they started to understand that there was something out there that affected their lives, yet they also realized that if they remained united, no harm would befall them.

The great ball of light was happy to see the sparks of light learned that they could indeed live alone but that they were also connected and could help each other. They learned that when they were united, even a very powerful force could not hurt them. He decided that each one of the balls of light was a family in and of itself, and all the sparks of light that existed within the family were brothers who must take care of each other. The size of the family was determined at the time of the bang and it could not be changed. A ball of light that contained ten sparks of light would remain with ten sparks of light, and a ball of light created with thousand sparks of light would remain with these thousand sparks of light.

Life within each of the balls flowed naturally. The sparks scampered around, got to know each other, and were happy with what they had.

Following this period of adjustment, the great ball was thinking about what to do with them: "I have realized what I wanted," he pondered. "I awakened my children, and they are alive. I provided them with all they need. They are relaxed, peaceful, and live in great order. Yet something is missing, something bothers me. All these sparks of light were created from me; I can see my spark in each and every one of them. Yet my spark within them does not give off light; it is dormant and inactive. There is no meaning to my spark which resides in each one of my children." He looked at his children and great warmth emanated from within him. This prompted him to continue ruminating: "I love them, they fill me with warmth, yet what should I do with them? What is the purpose of having created them?"

After observing himself for a moment, he understood: "The purpose of creating them is to produce more like me. I created countless children, and each one of them contains a part of me, the divine spark. Yet the spark hidden within them is dormant. The first thing I must do is awaken the divine spark within them."

The great ball brought all the balls of light close to him, as if he was embracing all of them together, and shot a purple ray of light that penetrated with great precision each one of the sparks of light. It was a spectacular sight. A purple source of light was turned on in each of the sparks. The sparks of light were excited by the sudden display and the change that overcame them.

The great ball let go of his embrace and stepped back. He looked at his children and was satisfied: "I awakened all the divine sparks hidden in each one of my children." After several moments of enjoyment, the shiny and sparkling sources of light gradually started to fade. The great ball failed to understand why. He immediately withdrew into himself in order to find the explanation for the unexpected event.

He needed some moments of self-observation in order to realize that as long as his children remained trapped within balls of light and did not have the freedom and independence he enjoyed, the divine spark latent in them was meaningless. "It is very easy to ignite the divine spark latent in each one of my children, yet in order to keep it burning they must use it. At this time, my children do not need to use the divine spark because I provide them with all their needs. Hence, I must grant freedom to my children, just like I have," he understood.

He was greatly saddened because he wanted them to always remain close to him, within the pleasant family cell he created for them. Yet at the same time he understood that should he continue providing all his children's needs, and should the family live only with itself, perfect harmony would prevail, so that none of the family members would feel a need to change or do anything. Everything would remain the same. However, this is what he wished to avoid more than anything else. He wanted his children to be well, yet not at any price. He took some time to think about how he could refrain from undermining their tranquility while still igniting the divine spark that existed in each and every one of them and keep it burning. After spending a lot of time thinking, he realized that there was no other choice; he must grant each one of his children freedom and independence. This was the only thing that would prompt the spark within them to awaken and act.

He set his objectives regarding his children:

"The noblest purpose is to awaken the divine spark that exists in each one of my children.

An additional goal is to grant each one of my children the opportunity to keep the divine spark burning, shining, and to get the most out of it."

Before acting, he thought about what this awakened divine spark would give each of his children. He was not sure whether he should infringe upon their serenity.

Within the spark exists the ability and potential to be free in all respects, the ability to be everywhere simultaneously, the ability to be boundlessly creative, the ability to influence, the ability to love, the ability to believe, the ability to persist, the ability to contain abundance of any kind, the ability to show compassion, the ability to feel a sense of belonging, the ability to rejoice, the ability to be brave, the ability to be vigorous, the ability to be passionate, the ability to be patient, the ability to be hopeful, and the ability to accept.

The great ball hesitated for a few more days. He felt sadness and loneliness over being exclusively responsible for his children and the only one that could make decisions for them. And then, he made a decision! The great ball of light straightened up and let out an immense roar that penetrated each of the balls. It was the first time they ever heard a sound. They were scared and once again converged into one unit, as if embracing each other, unmoving. The huge roar was followed by absolute quiet; still nobody moved. The great ball then started to speak to them:

"My dear, beloved children, I have never before addressed you directly and this is the first time you hear a voice of any kind. Have no fear; I am your father. You indeed cannot see me, yet you can certainly hear me, and you have already felt me in the past. I am the one who gave you life; you were created from me. I am the one who disturbs your peace now and I was the one who disturbed it in the past with powerful gusts of wind. Yes, it is I who created you. You are sparks of light within a ball of light and there are many like you. You are in different places and come in different sizes and colors, yet all of you are my children and I love you all."

The great ball grew silent. All the sparks within all the balls remained united, yet they let off some tension and relaxed a little. They sensed a pleasant warmth in his voice; they felt enveloped and waited for the voice to address them again. When the great ball saw that all of them were relaxed and tranquil, he continued:

"My dear, beloved children, my spark is contained in each one of you. Indeed, it exists, yet is dormant. I want the best for you, and as I am responsible for you, I have decided that I am obliged to awaken my spark, which exists in each one of you. This is my greatest mission.

I turn to you, my beautiful and wise creatures; you have tranquility, calm, pleasantness, and even company. However, my dear children, I am a father to all of you, I love you more than anything else, and I decided that at this time the most important thing for each one of you is freedom.

At this time, you live within a ball of light that constitutes a small family unit for you, yet I created many similar balls of light. The moment you gain freedom, you shall come out of your ball of light and meet me, as well as others from other balls."

The great ball had trouble letting go of his children. He spoke while large tears flowed from him like rain, making all the sparks of light feel cold.

"My dear, beloved sparks, freedom shall lead you to paths of life where the same harmony you have become accustomed to will not always be maintained. You are about to live independently. Only then will you be able to choose whether you wish to keep the divine spark inside you burning. You must understand, dear ones, that this is your choice. I wish to grant this golden opportunity to each one of you, and therefore I have decided to release you all. Whoever so wishes will be granted all the strength needed to awaken the divine spark and keep it burning. It pleases me to see that all of you are well and peaceful, yet it will please me even more to see you using the special spark within you."

The great ball continued to talk and explain to them while they listened to his words without moving. Eventually, he concluded:

"I want to explain to you what this spark I'm giving you is all about: It grants you independent lives. At this time you are controlled by me. If I exhale in your direction, you fly, and if I send you warmth, you grow warmer. You are indeed alive, yet you have no control over your lives. I gave you life and I am the one who controls it. My objective in creating you is to create a countless number of beings like me. I am completely independent, I exclusively control my own life, I determine my life path, I experience boundless creativity, I belong to all, and I can be anywhere simultaneously. I experience love, abundance of any kind, and freedom of any kind. All of this exists in each one of you, in your divine spark, and will have meaning should you keep your divine spark awake."

Everyone was silent. They drew apart from each other, moved closer again, united, and drew away again. They thought to themselves, "What will happen? On the one hand, meeting this father is intriguing, yet what shall happen if we go free?"

The great ball that can be anywhere simultaneously heard the inner conversations of all the sparks of light and responded to them:

"My dearest ones, you have something I do not have: you have a family unit you belong to, and you have my constant providence. You were created within a ball of light along with other sparks of light. You shall always belong to the same ball and you shall always be able to receive support and help from the other sparks of light that belong to your ball. At the same time, I shall always observe you, guide you, and protect you in times of need."

Everyone relaxed and the great ball left them to live for another period with the knowledge that something was about to change.

The great ball now had time to think and plan how to free his children from the balls of light and grant them independent lives.

First, he organized the balls. They were spread across a huge space, and he put them together into a pyramid structure. He organized them according to size and color. He placed the small balls containing a small quantity of sparks of light at the bottom of the pyramid, and as the quantity of sparks of light in each ball was larger, their position in the pyramid was higher. The great ball was at the top of the pyramid.

The great ball decided that once released, the sparks of light would spread to different areas, so that they would never meet. He wanted them to explore this journey independently and not be influenced so strongly by their family unit. He knew that should they meet, they would attempt to return to the ancient family unit, and rely only on each other instead of keeping the divine spark awake and eliciting all the goodness it offered. This would cause their inner power, their divine spark, to fade.

The debate was a difficult one. The great ball of light continued to ponder and sought the best path for his children.

"I want to see my children growing, developing, and creating. I want them to be like me, without boundaries and with powers of creation. Should they remain by my side as units of light they will not be able to grow and develop because they already have everything.

That being the case, the objective is for them to create a life of their own, a world of their own, exactly like the one I created for myself. I am about to grant my children independence and freedom of choice. They will be their own creators, and I will no longer hold exclusive influence over them."

He understood that in order to realize this objective, he must release them and *make them more sophisticated*. He must grant them something that he did not have.

At that moment of understanding, the great ball was overcome by incredible emotion and strength; he started to create millions of vessels. It was important for him to know how his children would feel, and therefore he tried all the vessels on himself.

Until one day, he came up with an idea: A highly sophisticated vessel comprised of three bodies: a physical body, a mental body—consciousness—and an energetic body. He decided to grant this masterpiece to his children.

Now, the great ball had to decide in which of the bodies he would place his sparks of light. He attempted to live within each one of the bodies, and when he entered the energetic body for the first time, he felt most comfortable; he felt at home.

Every day, he upgraded each one of the bodies; he polished and improved them, assigned them roles, and attempted to live within all kinds of life combinations: He lived with one body alone, he lived with two bodies, he modified their roles and created new roles for them, until he came up with the winning combination. It was a masterpiece that only he, the great ball, could create, and he called it "Man": a combination of three bodies—a physical body, a mental body, and an energetic body. He would place his sparks of light, his children, within the energetic body, hidden and invisible.

The great ball lived within the "Man" for a long period of time, examining and scrutinizing his creation, until he reached the conclusion: "I feel comfortable within the vessel known as 'Man.' I feel wonderful within the energetic body. I have plenty of space and room for expression, and I can certainly continue to be me and to function. The other two bodies limit me. It is not like just being pure light. On the other hand, they also safeguard and protect me."

He felt that if he was going to send his children far away from him, he must send them away protected and safeguarded. He did not want the precious thing he had created to be vulnerable, and it was no less important for him that all the qualities of light inherent in his masterpieces be preserved.

Following lengthy contemplation, he decided: "My children will not stay near me and will not remain like me, just light. They will live within the 'Man' I have created for them. It is better for them to be somewhat limited but protected. This way I shall be at peace with myself, knowing I did the best thing for them. I granted them absolute freedom within a limitation called 'Man.' They are my children, I created them, they are part of me, and the most important thing for me is to see them and their divine spark safeguarded."

Another dilemma, which was just as weighty, was where to place his children. Eventually he decided: "I must remove them from me and from the ball of light they belong to. That way, I shall grant them the opportunity to make use of the divine spark that exists within them."

He created another world: this world we live in.

And so, the great ball created the separation between the higher worlds and this world.

Chapter 3

Setting the Sparks of Light Free

The great ball was delighted with his masterpiece, "Man," with this world, and most of all, he was delighted to know that soon his children would be set free. He embraced all the balls of light in one big hug, and then it all started.

He exhaled powerfully from the top of the pyramid, spinning each one of the balls in a circular motion.

The sparks of light felt that something was moving them and understood that something was about to happen. They were even waiting for it. The great ball roared loudly, making each one of the balls tremble. The sparks of light stood still, and the great ball started to talk to them:

"My dearest children, the moment of truth has arrived. I have decided to start the journey towards independence by choosing the first balls from which sparks of light will be released. The sparks from these balls shall be set free simultaneously and descend to the new world I created.

This world is divided into various zones and you will be spread across them. Sparks of light that lived in the same ball of light shall not descend to the same zone. This separation will prevent you from meeting in this world.

Even though you shall not meet or see each other in this world, you can still be affected by each other. Your brothers who remain in the higher worlds, within your original balls of light, shall observe you and always be willing to offer their help.

Only from the purple and blue colored balls positioned right below me, will I release all the sparks of light simultaneously. They shall not descend to this world, but rather, stay with me and help me.

The other sparks that I will release shall descend from the higher worlds to this world via a tube of light that will come out of your ball of light and connect directly to this world. The color of the tube matches the color of the ball you are in, so that if the color of your ball is green, you shall come down to this world in a green colored tube.

The process of descent shall take seven of this world's days, and on the seventh day, you shall come out of the tube into this world. At the moment of discharge, you shall be present in a new world; you shall enter the masterpiece I created, called 'Man,' and you shall be born. The tubes that served you in passing from the higher worlds to this world will remain connected to your source, so that in any given moment you will be able to connect to your tube and receive light, love, and support both from the ball of light where you originated and from me.

The supreme objective of your existence in this world is to keep your divine spark awake and to use it."

From that moment, a process of internal preparation got underway in all the selected balls of light. The sparks of light chose who among them would descend to this world first.

In a flash, the great ball of light emitted a white light beam that simultaneously penetrated all the balls of light, indicating that the process had begun. The sparks of light came out of the balls of light and gathered in an orderly manner by their respective ball, waiting for further instructions from the great ball. The sight was spectacular and powerful, such that human eyes cannot bear. The entire space filled with magnificent, blinding lights.

The great ball spun around each of the sparks of light, penetrated them, and bestowed his presence, power, and strength upon them. He whispered his blessing to each one of them, and a moment later all the sparks of light waiting by the balls of light were sucked into the tube of light and were carried off, like a maelstrom, in the direction of this world. For seven days, the sparks of light went through a journey from the higher worlds to this world. They felt that they were being sucked within a fast, powerful spiral, until on the seventh day they were discharged from the tube into this world. At the moment of discharge, they entered the masterpiece known as "Man" and embarked on a new life.

The great ball divided his masterpiece, "Man," into males and females, and while inserting the sparks of light into the masterpiece, he made sure to have a balance between the genders; that is, half of them would be females, and half would be males.

During the first days in this world, they walked around hunched and withdrawn from the world. They lived as separate units; they did not look up and did not notice that there were others like them. They kept on walking with no defined purpose and occasionally returned to their tube and connected to the source from which they arrived. Through the tube, they were filled up with love and light. They sighed with relief and went back to their new daily routine in this world. They took pleasure in the wonderful sensations that the divine spark granted them; feelings of love, freedom, happiness, courage, hope, security, comfort, tranquility, vigor, passion, belonging, acceptance, patience, and compassion. As the days passed and the divine spark kept burning within them, they started to raise their heads and explore their new world.

Each day became more interesting than the previous. Each one of them was only preoccupied with himself or herself and with the wonderful sensations the spark aroused in them.

The sparks of light that came to this world into the masterpiece known as "Man" were henceforth known as "human beings." Life in this world became very active. The higher worlds and this world were separated, yet the connection of each human being to the place he or she arrived from, their origin, remained, and the great ball bestowed his love and presence upon everyone.

The human beings enjoyed life in this world and their connection to the higher worlds. Everyone possessed the inner knowledge that they were the great ball's children and that they were here in order to make use of the divine spark burning within them.

The moment the divine spark was awake within them, they were like the great ball and could do things the way he could. They started to use the powers inherent in the divine spark; they created on a daily basis, were at several places at the same time, maintained contact with the higher worlds and with this world, listened to themselves, and operated in line with an inner voice that guided them. They invented new things that served them, looked up and took notice of more masterpieces like them, met with them, spoke to them, shared, and helped each other. They lived a life full of freedom of choice, inspiration, and a plethora of goodness. The more they created, shared, helped, loved, and were joyous, the stronger the spark became, turning into a powerful, significant guide in their lives.

Yet there were some among these human beings who chose not to use the power hidden within their divine spark. They enjoyed what it gave them, yet did not preserve it through action, and so it kept on fading away until it almost completely disappeared.

The great ball watched his children from above and could not believe what he was seeing. He could not believe that some of his children were choosing not to do anything with the spark. His love for his children was so immense that he decided to send a powerful beam of light that would reignite their divine spark. Yet it was to no avail; they again chose to enjoy what the spark gave them without doing a thing with it, and the spark again faded away.

The great ball was saddened and realized that this was the price of freedom of choice, and that each one of his children was permitted to choose his own life path.

Life in the higher worlds continued to be managed in an exemplary manner, yet the simultaneous life in this world started to go awry. The divine spark faded among those human beings who chose not to preserve it, and they started to feel the opposite sensations of what they felt when the spark burned. They felt sadness, pain, boredom, frustration, fear, lack of belonging, loneliness, and other sensations which they had not experienced previously and which had not existed in the world.

It was the end of the "early days" era.

This world was divided into people of darkness and people of light. The people of light were human beings who chose to preserve the divine spark, so it kept on growing stronger within them, while the people of darkness were human beings who chose not to preserve the divine spark, and it faded away.

When the people of light were the majority, the effect on this world was positive, yet with the passage of time, there were more people of darkness, and chaos started to take root in this world. Human beings experienced feelings they had never felt until then, such as anger, sadness, helplessness, and despair. These feelings also started to affect the others around them. The state of this world was becoming unbalanced, and so the great ball felt he must intervene. At first he dispatched some of the sparks of light that remained by him. Remember them? He sent some of the purple and blue colored sparks of light, those that were next to him in the pyramid, ordering them to descend to this world so that the balance of light would be restored. This worked for a while, yet large quantities of darkness were created again. He sent down more sparks of light from the higher worlds to this world, yet among them there were some who chose not to use his divine spark, and with the passage of time the darkness grew and spread.

Although his greatest mission was indeed taking shape and some human beings were choosing to use the powers inherent in the divine spark, the great ball wondered what he should do with those who did not. He thought to himself, "There must be a way for me to bring all human beings to the point where, out of their own accord, they choose to preserve the divine spark within them and keep it burning throughout their lives."

Chapter 4

Joint Journey of Creation

As the great ball tried to find a solution for the state of this world, he started to receive inquiries from the people of light, asking to return to the higher worlds. Their main argument was that despite their ability to remain connected to the higher worlds, they were not satisfied and they longed for their homes, their origin in the higher worlds. They felt they no longer had anything to do in this world.

The number of inquiries kept growing, and the great ball decided this was not a bad solution: "We shall bring anyone who feels he made the most of himself in this world, as well as the human beings who chose not to make use of the divine spark, back to the higher worlds."

From that moment, a procession of coming and going got underway, and the sparks of light returned to their homes, yet not all at once. In order to maintain balance and order, every time one spark of light returned to its origin, that is, to its ball of light in the higher worlds, another spark of light came down to this world.

Those who returned to the higher worlds spoke of this world back home; they spoke about the difference between this world and the higher worlds, about the development of this world, about the people of darkness and people of light, about what they would have liked to change or add, and about all their personal experiences. Their brothers, who had watched them from the higher worlds, listened to them and guided them. Those returning to the higher worlds reported their actions in this world and made requests for the future. When they returned to the higher worlds, they possessed broader awareness. And so, if they started as identical sparks of light, as equal brothers, *their ability to choose and their actions in this world expanded their awareness.*

All the information about their lives in this world was relayed to the great ball. He received everything eagerly and addressed every request or question that came up.

Thousands of years passed and differences were created among the sparks of light. Some of them possessed broad awareness, while others possessed less. The great ball understood that things could not go on like that. His objective was for his children to develop and grow. He decided that a spark of light that made an effort and developed in this world would be promoted to a higher developmental stage in the higher worlds; that is, such a spark would change its color and location, so that from then on he would belong to a higher developmental group in the pyramid. And this indeed materialized. Sparks of light went up and down between the two worlds at an amazing rate. Every spark of light that returned to the higher worlds underwent a process where it recounted what it experienced and learned in this world. The great ball then associated the spark with the suitable developmental group in the higher worlds, a group that could contribute to the spark's development.

The great ball's solution of bringing up and sending down sparks of light, thereby boosting the balance of light in this world, only worked for a short period of time. The sparks of light that descended to this world again included some that chose not to make use of their divine spark, and so it faded away.

The great ball decided to impose a *restraint*. From that moment on, no sparks of light would descend to this world, yet sparks of light would continue to return to the higher worlds. He called it a *"cessation of descending souls."*

The great ball thought to himself, "What's happening to my children? They choose not to make use of all the abilities inherent in the incredibly special spark found within them, and on top of this, they do not even make an effort to preserve it!"

"It's impossible that they would choose to hurt themselves. Apparently, something is missing for them in this world. But what?" He recalled all the requests submitted by his children upon their return from this world to the higher worlds and noticed that many of them complained of longing for the family unit in the higher worlds.

The great ball understood that they lacked the close family ties they were accustomed to in the higher worlds. After all, as you may recall, in the higher worlds each and every one of the sparks of light belongs to a supportive, understanding, and loving family unit. They are always in touch with their brothers and are willing to offer help, even when they are not next to each other. The connection is uninterrupted, with no limits or obstacles.

He understood this and wanted to create a similar living environment in this world. The decision was to create family units. He connected female and male human beings, and was happy to see that they were showing an interest in each other. Harmony, care, concern, and absolute cooperation between the males and females were created.

Order started to take root in this world. Human beings who in the past chose not to use the divine spark and not to preserve it saw in their partner, whose spark was burning, something else—a better life—and were convinced to also arouse the spark found within them. They built joint, harmonious homes. The divine spark burned in each one of these human beings, and therefore it also burned in their homes.

The divine spark continued to burn in human beings and as time passed, it grew and became stronger.

Moreover, a new will awoke in them, a powerful desire to create life. Many couples turned to the great ball and asked to be given this opportunity.

The great ball was happy to hear of their desire and formulated a plan. "This moment was worth waiting for," he thought, "This is the greatest thing I could have wished for myself. They are asking me to enable them to create life on their own. Finally, it will be possible to put an end to the 'cessation of descending souls.' The life they shall create will be souls that come down from the higher worlds to this world. They shall come down according to a special request by the spouses in this world and based on my comprehensive examination of each spouse. And so, we shall see a correlation between the parents' request and the soul they receive."

The message was conveyed to everyone during their sleep. The great ball entered each human being, both the males and females, and informed them of the news that they can create life together:

"You are my children; I created you and brought you down to this world via a tube of light. You were discharged from the tube and entered the masterpiece known as 'Man.' In creating your own children you are full partners, and hence, the sparks of light known as souls will indeed descend from the higher worlds via a tube. Yet unlike you, they will not be directly discharged from the tube to this world, but rather, they shall pass through the female.

The tube shall come down from the ball of light of your offspring directly into the female's abdomen, to a place called the womb. Your offspring shall stay in the womb for nine moons, and through our joint cooperation, life shall be created. After nine moons, they shall be discharged from the womb into this world just like you were discharged from your tube of light. You are full partners, and therefore you hold responsibility and far-reaching influence over this masterpiece.

The female will carry the spark of light within her, to serve as a vessel and to provide it love, warmth and an existential security that until now only I was capable of providing.

The light that arrives from the higher worlds grants life to the spark of light contained in the womb. Without this light, the spark cannot develop and form life, and I therefore pledge to grant light from the higher worlds, as well as my constant protection, to those who hold life in their womb. This gift will make the divine spark burn powerfully in any female who holds life in her, passing on its power and strength to the spark held in the womb.

Another female role is to serve as a *transition vessel for* the human being formed inside her—transition from the womb to independent life in this world. The masterpiece known as 'Man' is to be discharged from the female just like she had been discharged from the tube of light into this world, and so at this stage she serves as a tube of light for her own masterpiece. The more open the tube is, the easier it is for her masterpiece to come out. This is to be an excellent period in her life where she can experience new life. The females have an effect on the lives of these sparks from the moment they enter the womb to the day they leave this world and return to the higher worlds.

The male is required to protect his family, and to provide the family with both physical and energetic food from the higher worlds. As opposed to the female, who receives the light effortlessly as a gift from the heavens, the male must work hard in order to pull the light down.

The male should not rely only on what the great ball gives; he must also acquire and aspire to receive as much light as possible from the higher worlds and pass it on to his family. The male's objective is to make his divine spark greater, through its daily usage as well as by pulling light from the higher worlds. When the male's divine spark burns, he enjoys the wonderful sensations provided by the spark; feelings of love, freedom, joy, courage, hope, self-confidence, comfort, tranquility, vigor, passion, belonging, acceptance, compassion, and patience. The male grants all of this to his partner in order to safeguard the life she is forming inside her."

The sparks of light woke up in the morning with new awareness! They were capable of creating life!

This marked the beginning of a magical, extraordinary journey.

The great ball created in the higher worlds a place that was home to all the sparks of light waiting to be summoned by human beings from this world. The sparks were waiting for a specific invitation, made especially for them, which would facilitate their release from the higher worlds into this world. They knew that they must wait patiently both for the specific invitation and for the examination by the great ball of their suitability for those who summoned them. Endless requests for creating life were coming from everywhere in this world where human beings resided. Everyone wanted to be a partner in creating life, everyone wanted to be like the great ball, and they each sent their request to the heavens. The great ball looked at all the requests and approved all of them. Sparks of light came down and each took root in the specific womb to which it was summoned and for which it was suitable.

A new life journey began, where human beings were part of the creation of life. The great ball knew that by doing this he was shifting further responsibility to these parents; responsibility he was bearing on his own shoulders until then. These human beings not only became responsible for themselves, but also assumed responsibility for each other, and together assumed responsibility for the masterpiece they were creating.

The life in the womb began. The sparks of light descended to the womb and started to receive life. The spouses had their own role and the great ball had his role. Both the great ball and the spouses took part in creating this life.

In every female who held life within her something burned, intensified. The light that flowed into her without any effort on her part prompted her divine spark to burn at full force and bestowed wonderful feelings upon her.

The female and the life within her became one. They felt each other and were affected by each other. Members of the female gender were responsible for safeguarding themselves—their three bodies—and for supplying material food to the sparks of light that developed within them. All the females, with no exception, fulfilled their life mission. Moreover, they felt a great commitment and an immense sense of love for the life being formed within them, so although the great ball provided them with light without requiring any effort on their part, they felt they needed to connect to the higher worlds on a daily basis and pull light into themselves.

This period became an amazing, dynamic era. Members of both the female and male genders shared in the process of nurturing the new life inside the female. They took part in this mission together. The divine sparks burned with great force within everyone, and all human beings made the most of their divine spark.

After nine moons, a miraculous process took place. A human being came out of the female womb. Everyone was overjoyed. The parents decided that they were assuming full responsibility for their child with respect to his or her life here in this world. With all the love they felt, their heart kept growing, and it was as if it had not existed before. Suddenly they started to feel immense love enveloping them. The great ball watched on from above and was elated. He even laughed. "They feel what I feel towards them. What a masterpiece!" he said with great satisfaction.

The great ball gave the newborn baby a gift. He decided that in addition to the protection granted by him and the parents, he would provide the newborn baby with yet another protection, a "higher guidance." This guidance would accompany the baby throughout his entire life. The higher guidance would stay in the higher worlds, yet when necessary it would come down and help him in this world. The great ball also decided that this guidance would change in accordance with the person's actions and his level of development in this world.

The mother, too, received a gift from the great ball. While giving birth, she was cleansed of her past as if she were reborn.

The birth experience was wonderful both for the female and for the tiny human who had just been discharged from her womb. The male was overcome by love and amazement, expressing his gratitude to the great ball and to his spouse for the great miracle that occurred in his life. The tiny human had a mother and father in this world, and a father in the higher worlds.

The newborn baby was happy and was enveloped by an amazing sense of security. Everyone around the baby loved him, and he felt protected. All the children were connected to both worlds and enjoyed nourishment from both.

The parents learned the needs of the newborn baby. They fed, played with, and taught their baby, while embracing him with love. Every day, they expressed their gratitude to the great ball for the incredible gift they received. Life continued normally, and all human beings were content and possessed an abundance of everything.

Ever since children began to arrive in the world, the balance of light increased considerably, and life in this world changed completely. Human beings went back to living the way they used to live in the "early days" era. The ties among human beings grew stronger, they felt a sense of commitment and mutual responsibility, their ability to give grew, their capacity to sympathize with others became stronger, and family units were created. Time passed and the first children who arrived through the womb took part in creating their own masterpieces. It was a wonderful period. The number of human beings in this world kept growing, and the great ball took pleasure in the natural development that took place and the incredibly strong ties created in this world.

At the beginning of every month, representatives of each family would gather for a meeting in order to discuss various issues. At one of the meetings, the topic was "Children and Their Connection to the Higher Worlds." Children of various ages were summoned to this session and spoke about their lives. They spoke of their immense desire to be connected to the higher worlds and of the great ease with which they created this connection. They also described the magnificent feeling and connection they had experienced since the day of their birth with their higher guidance, which was providing them with answers to many questions. They also spoke of how happy they were with what they possessed and how their lives were filled with positivity, creativity, love, happiness, health, and a connection to their inner selves and to the higher worlds.

At the end of this meeting, one of the children stood and thanked the parents on behalf of all the children:

"Dear parents, we are grateful to you for enabling us to experience a full, harmonious life. Every day since the day we were born, we see, experience, and feel your presence. We emulate your behavior and imitate with great accuracy the language you speak. We also emulate your innermost thoughts, so that even if you do not express them aloud, we hear and see them via our highly developed inner senses. We do not miss any blink, any wrinkle of laughter, or any tear. Everything goes through us, and we are a part of your lives regardless of our age and location. We always feel you and are aware of what you are experiencing. We thank you for the abundance we have in our lives, for your limitless love, and for the connection with the higher worlds. We thank you and love you with no limits."

The children left and complete silence prevailed! Nobody spoke. Some wiped away tears of joy, while others sat there and waited. Everyone raised their heads to the great ball and thanked him for enabling them to take part in the creation of life.

Each one of those present sat upright, ensured that his tube was connected to the higher worlds, and pulled an incredible quantity of light of different colors, so that the space was filled with a myriad of spectacular colors. A sense of relaxation and tranquility filled the place.

Time was dedicated for everyone to be with himself. During that time, each person concentrated on himself and thought positive thoughts about himself and his family. Shortly after, the discussion continued.

Towards the end of the discussion, various representatives spoke about what they experienced while being with themselves. One representative spoke of meeting his dear spouse who had returned to the higher worlds. He embraced her and shared what he was going through. From her he received guidance and recommendations regarding his personal development and this strengthened him very much. Another person shared with the audience the magical journey he had been drawn into; a journey below the fertile earth that revives us[2].

The conclusion of the meeting was as follows:

> "Parents have a far-reaching influence on their children from the moment they take root in the womb to the day they return to the higher worlds, regardless of their age and location."

They all bid each other farewell and left the meeting satisfied and happy with what they had and overjoyed knowing that their children imitate their positive behavior, whether consciously or unconsciously. They knew that this was being passed on even without words!

Many years passed. Many lives were created in this world, and great joy prevailed. As long as the divine spark burned and operated within each of the souls, life was harmonious and good.

---

[2] You will learn more about this and other healing techniques in a subsequent book

Chapter 5

The Children Get Hurt

Every day, transparent bubbles that contained the divine light were being sent to this world. They were buried in the ground and created peace and tranquility in this world. Everyone enjoyed the gifts sent by the great ball.

An immense change had occurred in this world; everyone had become united. The divine spark burned in all of them. All homes were filled with glee, laughter, and love. Something in everyone's heart had opened up and expanded. Families were connected in one circle and did not want it to be broken.

Peace and tranquility prevailed until the day came when one of the parents completed his role in this world and had to return to the higher worlds. Yet unlike previous times, this time the matter was more complex. If in the past the return of a soul to the higher worlds was perceived as a routine, commonplace, and daily event, it was now perceived as undesirable and painful. Human beings no longer lived as separate units or as couples. The children, the masterpieces they took part in creating, entered their lives and made them completely different.

The moment the children arrived in this world, ties at home became tighter and more powerful, and now it was very difficult to part. Each member of the family felt a sense of belonging and great love, and each wanted this state of affairs to continue. The children wanted their parents, and the parents felt love and responsibility for their children and did not wish to leave.

At first, the great ball did not understand what the fuss was all about. Everything was planned and orderly; some souls come down and others go up. Yet in the eyes of human beings, things were being perceived in a wholly different manner. Great cries resonated from this world to the great ball, cries and pleas for him to keep everyone in this world. The families felt very united; they depended on each other and did not wish to separate. The great ball saw that his children were suffering and sent a widespread message to all the homes:

"My dear, beloved souls, remove any worry from your hearts. Some of you have to leave this world, yet those who leave will be with those who stay at any given moment, even when they are in the higher worlds. All you have to do is keep your divine spark burning, and this will enable you to be in both worlds simultaneously."

The children sent him a message in response: "We do not agree and do not want to separate from our parents; we want them here with us forever."

The great ball responded:

"My dear children, it is impossible for all the parents to stay here. Some of the parents no longer have anything to do here. If they stay nonetheless, their divine spark shall keep on fading and they shall experience very difficult lives."

The great ball understood the children's feelings yet he knew that despite the sense of loss, the turnover of souls ensured that their divine spark would keep burning and benefit them. He then offered extensive help and brought down light and love to all homes in order to help human beings overcome the sense of loss. Many homes reconciled themselves to the situation and understood that this was the right thing to do. Yet some homes strongly rebelled. These homes severed their ties with the higher worlds and immense anger accumulated against the great ball.

They complained: "Why don't you bring all the souls from the higher worlds down here? Why do you take us back to you? We do not wish to return; we feel good here with our family."

The great ball responded immediately and provided an explanation:

"My dear children, I understand how you feel, yet I want to explain to you several things. Some of you exhausted your life's mission and need to return to the higher worlds. Moreover, to my surprise, at the very start of your journey in this world there were those of you who chose not to make use of the magnificent abilities inherent in the divine spark, and so it kept fading. This created the opposite feelings of those granted by the divine spark: weakness, lack of belonging, frustration, and more.

In this world, you are granted the freedom of choice. You choose how to live your lives and you are your own masters, yet you do not live in this world on your own. You affect and are affected by others, and for that reason I have no intention of bringing all the souls down and waiting to see what each one of them chooses to do. After all, it is possible that many of you would choose to do nothing with the divine spark. This choice would affect both those of you who choose not to use the spark as well as those who do wonders with the spark.

Hence, those who have not made use of their divine spark and those who have exhausted their life here in this world I will send back to the higher worlds. I will assign them a study group that fits their developmental level based on what they did in this world. In this group the person studies, develops, and is always willing to take part in helping this world."

Most families accepted the situation and understood that if the soul has completed its role here in this world, it should return to the higher worlds, to its origin and to its initial family that it missed. As long as understanding and acceptance of the situation prevailed, the families continued to live happy lives and maintained a direct contact with the higher worlds. They increased the size of their families and were happy with every miracle, every soul that descended from the higher worlds to their home.

Yet some of the families who experienced the loss did not reconcile themselves to this situation. They felt a sense of anger and bitterness towards the great ball.

The great ball addressed everyone with a clear message:

"My dear souls, I am not bothered by the anger you feel towards me. It even warms my heart to see how much you love each other. However, you are only hurting yourselves. *Every time you are angry towards me, you create negativity in your lives and thereby prompt your divine spark to fade.*"

Some of them accepted the message and immediately curbed their anger, yet others continued to be angry and hurt themselves. This saddened the great ball, and he again turned to all those human beings who had trouble accepting the loss:

"Kind, brave, dearest souls, remove negativity from your lives and bring the light into your homes. I am sending assistance from the heavens to your homes."

Immediately after the great ball had finished, purple colored light with silver sparks came down from the higher worlds and entered every home that contained negativity. The light that entered the homes immediately alleviated the situation and all the families reverted to a quiet, comfortable routine.

However, this period of relaxation did not last for long. Several days later, these same human beings were again angry towards the great ball. This time, their anger kept growing. As was previously the case, the great ball understood that he could not protect his children all the time and that they had to choose whether they would accept his help. He was always there to listen and offer his assistance, yet they needed to seek and want it.

Nothing helped. The divine spark within these human beings faded. These human beings walked around with negative feelings that were the opposite of what they sensed when their divine spark was burning. They experienced sadness, weakness, lack of belonging, frustration, solitude, anger, and more.

The human beings whose negativity became a significant part of their lives started to negatively affect their environment and suffered disruptions to various bodily systems. They found themselves facing situations of distress that did not exist in the world previously.

With the passage of time, more and more *adults* were suffering from various forms of distress and could not find a cure. Some of the families who lived positive lives attempted to offer their help, yet to no avail. Nothing prompted these parents to embark on renewed action and the creation of ties to the higher worlds. They remained "stuck" within their own bubble.

Initially, negativity spread only among the parents who chose to live negative lives, yet as time passed this was bearing down upon their children as well. The children of the negative parents experienced the negativity on a daily basis and it penetrated their lives. And so, even if they did not directly behave in a negative manner, they ate, drank, heard, and felt the negativity. This reality prompted suffering among the children as well, something which did not exist before. The fruit of the masterpiece, which was the greatest miracle of all, was harmed.

Many understood the gravity of the situation. They declared a state of emergency and dubbed the situation "the negativity epidemic." Moreover, they decided to convene an emergency meeting aimed at "eradicating the negativity epidemic from this world."

A message was conveyed to each home:

"Dear family,

You are hereby invited to an emergency meeting aimed at eradicating negativity from our lives. By the meeting date, each family is hereby requested to brainstorm about how to eradicate the epidemic."

Upon receiving the message, families got together and came up with ideas to rid this world of the epidemic. Each family sent a request to the higher worlds, asking for assistance in this world. An immense number of requests arrived at the higher worlds, and all of these requests included the same message: "Help us eradicate the negativity epidemic."

The meeting day arrived. When the meeting started the oldest soul in this world was invited to take the stage. He was a tall man with a white, long beard, a pure expression, and small, deep blue eyes. The oldest of souls had the privilege of commencing the meeting. He stood in front of the participants and all eyes were on him. The light radiating around him gave confidence and serenity to all. For many it was the first time they had ever met with such a pure soul.

The oldest of souls turned to the participants:

"Dear souls, we have reached an era where negativity is created around us."

The oldest of souls paused for a moment and then continued, "Yet those of us present do not live the negativity and therefore we do not have the inner desire to change it. After all, you know that if we had the desire for change within us, there would be nothing to stand in our way. We have everything we need. We have health, we have each other, and we have help from the heavens. You have indeed heard about the negativity and some of you have seen its effects, yet you have never experienced it. Therefore, we must experience the negativity first-hand. Then the desire to remove it from our lives will awaken within us."

The oldest of souls instructed everyone to close their eyes and think a negative thought of their choice about him. Everyone closed their eyes, yet had trouble implementing the instructions. They did not know how to do it. He explained to them that they should think the opposite of positive, for example: If someone wishes me peace at home, he should wish me the opposite.

Everyone simultaneously thought a negative thought about the old man. The power of the thought was passed on to him like a powerful electric current, directly into his chest, and he collapsed at once and remained there lifeless. Great panic ensued. Some froze in place, stunned. Only the old man's wife maintained composure. She stood up and looked at the audience. Complete silence prevailed.

"I understand your consternation," she said in a quiet, clear voice. "I ask all of you to close your eyes and think a positive thought about my dear spouse." Everyone quickly closed their eyes and thought positive thoughts about the oldest of souls. They blessed him and wished him all the best they could imagine. Shortly thereafter, they witnessed what they were hoping for yet did not believe possible. The old man, who just a moment earlier was lying there lifeless, stood up and quickly continued to speak as if nothing had happened.

"What we did here now was to deliberately convey negative thoughts. We had here incredible negative power directed at me, and this is why I collapsed. Yet in some situations negativity seeps into our lives gradually, affecting us and our entire lives. Indeed, the effect is gradual and at times invisible, yet it is most certainly damaging, and with time we shall suffer the same things suffered by those who chose the path of negativity."

Everyone was fascinated and a little scared. Their pupils became unusually enlarged. The old man decided to take a break for drinking, and each participant drank a glass full of pink light energy. They took pleasure in the drink and were again calm and relaxed. Once the old man felt everyone was calm, he continued:

"You understand that even if you have positivity interwoven into your lives, negativity prevails around you, and you and your relatives are affected by it. The whole environment is affected by it. The earth we live on, the crops we eat, the water we drink, and the physical body we use, they all become tainted by the negative.

Thus far, we have familiarized ourselves with the effects of negativity on a person and his environment. The effects touch upon all areas of life: suffering is created in the physical body; peace at home is breached; families experience misery. This is the information we possess, yet with the passage of time the epidemic spreads and becomes increasingly stronger; it seeps in and affects many areas of life in ways we are still unfamiliar with and cannot fathom.

Hence, we gathered here today in an attempt to eradicate the epidemic. Each family was asked to come up with a solution, and now I turn the time over to you."

The oldest of souls completed his speech. Each participant was given the right to speak and come up with ideas on how to eradicate the negativity. They then summarized the proposals:

- We shall learn more about the negativity epidemic and its effects on us, and by doing so, we shall be able to turn the negative into something positive and minimize the harm.

- We shall pull more light from the higher worlds and use it in all areas of life.

- Every day, each one of us shall perform five good deeds, two of them for strangers.

- We shall offer our help to others.

- We shall check whether negativity exists in our life, and if it does, we will eradicate it.

- Every day, we shall bless two human beings.

- We shall bless the food and the drink in order to remove the negativity from them.

- We shall focus on our own development and not compare ourselves to others.

- We shall assume responsibility and control over our actions and thoughts.

When everyone was done speaking, the oldest of souls addressed the audience:

"Dear families, all the ideas are excellent and we shall use all of them. These ideas can indeed help prevent the epidemic from spreading into our lives. Yet to my regret, the ideas are unsuitable for families where negativity is already part of their lives. Hence, we shall not be able to eradicate the epidemic using these ideas, but rather only moderate its spreading."

All the participants listened, yet did not quite understand in their hearts what the oldest of souls understood. The image of the oldest of souls collapsing as result of the negative thoughts directed at him kept resonating in their minds, yet they had never experienced negativity within themselves. They did not feel negativity on their "flesh," and hence they could not envision what might take place in the future. They therefore could not come up with a suitable solution.

The oldest of souls, on the other hand, possessed immense knowledge and extensive life experience. He was exposed on a daily basis to many human beings who lived negative lives and sought a cure for their condition. He treated many people in this world and corrected various life situations. He decided that he must open the eyes of all the participants to what was happening in the world and do so in a manner that would touch their hearts, so that they all would be compelled to eradicate negativity. However, he still did not know how to do it.

The oldest of souls closed his eyes and asked for help form the great ball, "Father, please help me. Give me a sign; show me what I should do." The old man remained introverted for a few moments, waiting for an answer from within.

When he opened his eyes, they fell upon a young boy in the audience. He was astonished by the boy's presence, as this was a meeting of only adults. The oldest of souls felt that the child's presence was not accidental, and his eyes glowed with joy. He signaled the child to approach him.

"What are you doing here, my child?"

-"I know that you are holding an emergency meeting on eliminating the negativity epidemic and I know I can help."

The oldest of souls looked into the eyes of the child, as if he was looking into his soul, and then responded, "Thank you for coming, son. I know that you can help." The old man turned his gaze to the audience and called out:

"Dear friends, our young guest is offering his help. The timing could not be better. I suggest that we listen to his words."

The participants nodded in agreement. They were hypnotized by the boy's incredible purity as he stood in front of them. He was a beautiful boy with red, silky hair. As he started to speak, his big blue eyes gazed upon them.

"I want to share the story of my life with you. When I was a toddler, my grandfather left this world. My father did not reconcile himself with the departure and ever since the entire family has been suffering. He thinks negatively and does negative things to my mother and to others around him. He yells at home and uses unpleasant words. This is starting to affect my brother and me. Until recently, we haven't performed any negative deeds deliberately; we did not know how to think that way. Yet we have become exposed to this phenomenon and I am sorry to say that we are starting to emulate our father's behavior, even without realizing it. I find myself yelling at my brother, and twice I even shoved him violently. The effect on us is so great that my young brother told me that he sensed my father' negativity back in the womb and this disturbed my brother's peace and even made his entry into this world more difficult."

"That's it!" the oldest of souls turned to the audience. "Many of us will not change in order to prevent suffering and even alleviate suffering in our own lives. But once our children get hurt, we will do whatever we can and will improve ourselves in order to uproot suffering in them. We must all understand the direct connection between our actions, thoughts, and deeds and our children's wellbeing."

The oldest of souls embraced the child and thanked him. He then quoted the children's message to the parents in the previous meeting:

"From the day we are born, we see, experience, and feel your presence. We emulate your behavior and imitate with great accuracy the language you speak. We also emulate your innermost thoughts, so that even if you do not express them aloud, we hear and see them via our highly developed inner senses. We do not miss any blink, any wrinkle of laughter, or any tear. Everything goes through us, and we're a part of your lives regardless of our age and location."

"Children are a reflection of their parents," the oldest of souls explained, "They are affected by every behavior and thought that exists in their living environment. They grow up with all the information that seeps in and is absorbed into them. If this information is negative, our children shall live and breathe negativity. Indeed, at this time positivity reigns and your children are safe and protected. Yet look around you and see how many human beings are suffering in this world. You need to understand that we are all inextricably tied. Thus with the passage of time, negativity will seep into our lives and through us to our children; it will seep through our children into their children. The effects will be destructive from the moment the children enter the womb."

"The situation is graver than what you can imagine," the oldest of souls warned. "Our children are about to be harmed. We must not be quiet and we must not remain asleep! We must wake up and assume collective responsibility."

Those present sat there agape. The possibility of their children and grandchildren getting hurt shocked them and awakened within them a strong will to do whatever it would take to eradicate the negativity epidemic.

"First of all," the oldest of souls explained, "you must all convey everything that came up in this meeting to your family members and to every family you know. Help families where negativity reigns to understand the implications of negativity that lies within them on their children and generations to come."

"And most importantly," the oldest of souls added, "each one of you must look into himself every day and find out whether there is negativity in your life. In order to eradicate negativity, we should engage in a constant process of self-examination and correction.

I love you all and believe that together we can make it happen."

~

I would like us to take a break and rest a little. I feel terrible tension; it was so pleasant before, yet suddenly this negativity came and has made it feel unpleasant.

In order to clear the air, let us engage in self-examination to determine whether negativity exists within our lives. The next exercise will enable you to identify negativity that might exist in yourself and remove it from your life.

Exercise: Taking Out Negativity

This exercise will acquaint you with your inner self. Once you bring to the surface all there is to cleanse and you start working on it, you will create a significant turning point in your life.

For this exercise, you need a pen, a notebook, an index card, and preferably a highlighter as well.

In order to perform this exercise properly, first read the whole exercise, and then perform it.

- Write down how you *produce* negativity. For example, by not keeping your promises, not expressing feelings, being jealous, judging others, criticizing, being managed by fears, holding a grudge, cheating, etc.

- Write down the ways in which you *express* negativity. For example, by screaming, arguing, hitting, lying, gossiping.

- Write down how the negativity you produce or express harms you.

- Write down how the negativity you produce or express harms others.

- Read what you wrote and highlight three negative things you choose to remove from your life.

- Observe each of the things you chose to remove from your life, and turn them into something positive.

When you turn something to positive, it does not mean it has to be the opposite from what you chose. If, for example, you chose to remove anger, it does not mean you need to choose to be "calm." You can choose, for example, to be "patient."

You basically *choose* who you want to be. Use the adjective form. Whatever you choose should complete the sentence "I choose to be..." For example, if you choose to turn anger into patience, write "*patient.*"

In order for this exercise to serve as a significant turning point in your life, it is important that you be accurate. In order to be accurate, you need to *observe yourself from outside and see how the thing you chose to remove comes into play in your life. Examine what you need to do or think in order for it not to be present in your life anymore.*

Let us examine a case in which two people choose to remove anger. Although it might seem they both need to work on the same thing, each of them expresses anger differently: one by screaming and losing control, and the other by keeping the anger inside, remaining quiet, shutting himself down and keeping distance. Each of these people expressed anger differently.

In each moment of our lives, we can choose the role we want to play. For example, if until now the first person was "nervous," today he chooses to be "restrained." The other person who until now was "reserved" will choose to speak up.

- Write on a new page the positive things you committed to do.

    For example, if you chose to remove from your life:

    Anger, jealousy, lack of organization

    You can select the adjectives:

    Restrained, loving, organized

- Copy to the index card all you committed to improve. For example:

    "I, Sylvia Jones (specify your full name), am

    Restrained

    Loving

    Organized"

How to Use the Index Card

I advise you to laminate the card and put it in your purse or wallet. Read the card four times each day.

Every morning, when you wake up, take a deep breath, express your gratitude for another day you received, and read the things you pledged. Only then, start your day.

Read again at noon, at 3 p.m. and at 6 p.m. If you are going out at night, read the card before going out.

Reading With Intention

Reading with intention is a type of reading in which the reader puts his meaning to whatever he reads. People can choose to be loving. The word love is immense and contains many things within it. In order to generate a significant turning point in your life and to change the things which waste so much energy and which hurt you and others, *it is not enough to read the word "love" to become loving.* You need to enter a new meaning to what you chose to be. *You have to insert who you want to be* into everything you chose.

I want you to visualize how the thing you chose to change is going to appear in your life. Choose something practical, visual, and measurable.

A good actor is one who goes on a stage and does not just read the script. He literally lives it. Similarly, if you choose to be loving, read "loving" with intention. When I read in the morning the word "loving," I mean that I commit to hug my children three times a day. On the other hand, someone else who chooses to be loving commits to listen to her spouse. A person who chooses to be restrained may commit to count to three before he reacts or formulate and organize his thoughts before speaking.

Keep in mind that those around you will continue to behave in line with their own patterns. Be patient. You are the one who has chosen to improve yourself, and hence, do not try to change others. Focus on yourself. A person who changes himself creates a change in his environment.

Stay with the same commitments until you feel they are part of you, and then commit to new things, using a new index card.

~~~

Pay attention to what you are saying, how you speak, and what kinds of thoughts go through your mind. Every time you notice a negative thought entering, cancel it. I will now teach you a technique that will help you do that.

Technique for Abolishing Negative Thoughts

Every time you notice a negative thought, a bothersome thought, or a negative inner conversation with yourself or with others, stop it immediately. Envision yourself removing it from your mind, say "Null and void" three times, and bless yourself or the person you thought negatively about: "blessed,

blessed..." Continue saying the word "blessed" *until the thought evaporates from your mind.*

If you are thinking about a negative scenario, stop the scenario, rewind it, envision yourself removing it from your head, say "Null and void" three times, and bless: "blessed, blessed..." Bless anyone who was present in your scenario, until it is erased from your mind.

With all the joy that accompanies the birth of one of your children, you, the parent, are also assuming great worries. Worries are indeed negative energy. You, as parents, have a far-reaching influence on your children, and therefore the concern and fear that something bad may happen to your loved ones is passed on to your children, affects them negatively, and may create the reality you so much fear.

The energy of concern comes as a thought or as an entire scenario. For example, a boy is standing on a chair. His mother may run an entire scenario in her head: she sees him falling down, suffering a concussion, sustaining brain damage, and being unable to speak. After all, such reality could happen, yet at the moment it is only imaginary. I ask that in such cases, you close your eyes and rewind the scenario to the point before something negative happened. In the example above, the mother rewinds the scenario to the point where the boy is standing on the chair. She then sees herself walking over to him, hugging him, and bringing him down to the floor. After rewinding the scenario, say "Null and void" three times and bless the person you thought about: "blessed, blessed, blessed…"

You may perform this technique dozens of times a day. It is important that you persist!

This technique for abolishing negative thoughts is a wonderful way to overcome negativity and to cleanse your consciousness. In the chapter "Cleansing the Mental Body," on page 162, we will learn a *CCH* Technique for abolishing negative thoughts.

Chapter 6

Returning to the "Early Days" Era

The last meeting led many to understand that the situation in this world had to change, and quickly, or else more and more children would be harmed. The negativity epidemic was spreading, and both children and adults enlisted in the cause of eradicating it. They devoted themselves to action aimed at eradicating negativity, they held lectures on the issue of negativity, and they examined the following questions, "What does negativity do to the world? What may it cause in the future? What is negativity's effect on life?" Support centers for families where negativity dominated were opened. Yet despite all these efforts, the epidemic was not yet eradicated.

In the negativity epidemic, some were actively ill and others passively ill.

Actively ill were all human beings who made negativity a part of their lives. They thought in a negative manner and performed negative acts.

Passively ill were all the ones who were exposed on a daily basis to the effects of the negative human beings. That is, the passively ill did not think or act negatively, yet the results of the negative actions of those around them affected them too, and with time caused them suffering. Mostly exposed to this form of passive effect were the children whose parents' thoughts and actions were passed on to them, whether consciously or not.

Many homes where negativity was part of everyday life did not wish to change a thing. Children in these homes were exposed to the passive effect. They breathed, ate, heard, and felt negativity and it seeped into them. With the passage of time, children experienced suffering and fetuses absorbed negativity in their mother's womb and were born into a reality of suffering. From the day of their birth, they experienced suffering, difficulty, and pain. Negativity seeped so deeply into their lives that it afflicted them with the active form of the illness. They thought negatively and performed negative acts.

Nobody remained indifferent to this state of affairs. Parents and grandparents could not bear to see the children suffering; their pain was great and they wanted with all their hearts to do whatever possible in order to extract negativity and suffering from the children's lives. Heartfelt cries were heard as the suffering was so great and intolerable. The intentions expressed in the cries were deeply focused, and the heavens complied quickly.

The great ball came down to this world and spread such an immense quantity of light that it froze life. The ongoing movement in this world came to a halt. The great ball entered each and every human being and conveyed the following message:

"It will not help you to seek my assistance every time your children suffer; the solution is found within you. You must eradicate the incredibly sick roots buried deep inside you. Your children are a mirror of yourselves. Do not ask who to blame for their condition and do not seek outside answers to why they are suffering, why they are undisciplined, why they suffer from attention deficit disorders, or why they do not behave politely.

All the answers are within you. Your children came to you based on your special order, they are suitable for your own personal development, and they come to awaken you to inner work. Everything they are and everything they shall be in the future is based on who you are and what you have instilled in them through your way of life and your personal motives. Look at them and see yourselves. Through them, you can understand what you need to correct and improve. Hence, if you wish to correct their situation, cleanse yourselves. By so doing you shall directly affect their lives."

The great ball finished speaking and set the world in motion once again. Everyone without exception woke up stunned by the extraordinary experience. Human beings were used to making use of the light in various dosages and frequencies, and so they each responded to the light differently. Some of them collapsed, others cried, and some breathed a sigh of relief. The light did wonders for babies and children and the suffering was immediately erased from their lives.

The human beings could not believe what they had heard. They approached each other on the street and shared their experience with excitement. Indeed, everyone had heard the same thing. Everyone was overwhelmed with emotion. It was the first time that all human beings, without exception, wanted to change, and wanted to remove negativity from their lives. They sought the help of the oldest of souls and he convened a meeting, which he referred to as "a return to the early days."

Everyone agreed it was important for the meeting to be successful and families started to prepare a month in advance. The goal was to find a cure for the epidemic. What made this meeting special was the cooperation of all families, *including the families where negativity reigned.* There was a feeling of celebration in the air, a feeling of hope and common will for a change.

The eagerly anticipated day arrived. Silence prevailed among the audience as the oldest of souls stood before them.

"As you all know, I'm accustomed to dreaming prophetic dreams. Many human beings approach me with questions and I, in most cases, dream the answers.

Throughout my life in this world, I have dreamt positive dreams, yet a few years ago, I dreamt a negative dream that left a dark spot in my heart. I did not know whether to attribute this dream to the universal situation whereby negativity had entered human life and had also entered mine, or whether it was one of those prophetic dreams. I did not share this dream with anyone, not even my dearly beloved spouse. Yet now is the time to share it with all of you.

In the dream I saw dark, dense wind reach our world. The wind carried immense power and erupted from the ground like a volcano, it came from the sea in a great storm, and it came down from the skies like a huge downpour. At first, it just spun at great speed but then in a flash, it started to penetrate you. It penetrated directly into your eyes and turned you into naysayers, seeing everything as dark.

I fought this powerful wind with all my might. I blew in your eyes powerfully, yet the wind settled in your eyes like tiny grains of sand; it clung to them and would not leave. I attempted to fight it time and again, yet the more I tried, the stronger it became, as if it was angered by my repeated attempts. The wind gradually veiled all the abundance and light that arrived from the higher worlds and left our world with distress and suffering. I had never known such a wicked force and I did not know how to contend with it."

Tears were streaming from the eyes of the oldest of soul's spouse, and her heart was pounding. She did not share with anyone that she also had the same dream.

The oldest of souls walked over to her and wiped away her tears. "Don't cry, my dearest. The great ball is here with us and he gave me a way to eradicate the epidemic." Everyone embraced and sent love to each other.

"I dream and pray day and night to return to those days which were filled with light; days where I and other souls were the first to live in this world. I pray for help from the higher worlds, and that each and every one of you shall experience a life of perfect harmony.

I am one of those first souls who came down from the higher worlds to this world, yet I never returned to the higher worlds. You have always known that I possess great knowledge. You have consulted with me and have respected my views. You have wondered how I looked so young despite being such an old soul and how I possess such great knowledge in so many different areas of life. There must have been many other questions that you have come up with and have never asked. Today the great ball has asked me to tell you who I am and to speak to you about the 'early days' era.

It was a period of life that was filled with love, vitality, and creativity. We had an abundance of everything and great accessibility to the higher worlds. The connection with the higher worlds was continuous throughout every day.

When the great ball decided that we would be granted independence, he explained to us that there was another world he had created, which is this world we live in. It is a parallel world to the higher worlds, but in this world we would have to create the things we needed. He also explained to us that he created us whole, in perfect health, that we are part of him, and that this privilege grants us the ability to be like him. All we have to do is keep the divine spark within us burning.

We descended to this world and all around us were giant dunes and pools of light of different colors and textures. Each color had its own meaning and role. For many days, we walked through the dunes of light, ate from them, and slept in them. Each one of us was with himself and with the dune he needed. We enjoyed the same abundance we had in the higher worlds. We possessed the light and it streamed to us in abundance.

During those days, we were fed by light alone, light of different colors based on our daily needs. We ate and drank light. After a period of adjustment, when the divine spark was burning inside us and we were awake and accustomed to the physical and mental body we received, more and more needs started to arise.

From that moment on, all the souls worked diligently and happily in order to create this world. Every day, we created everything that today is taken for granted. We turned to the great ball and he helped us with every request.

In fact, we copied from the higher worlds what we needed in this world.

You probably wish to know how this was done. We all worked in cooperation and with special focus on each creation. The great ball would come down from the higher worlds and guide us. We would express our desires and he would create it together with us. He was a full partner in our creations. He is a master thinker and creator! Through his abilities, we saw the abilities inherent in us and from him we learned that we, too, can create whatever comes to mind, using our willpower, our intention, and our focus. It was an extraordinary experience for all of us. We witnessed the greatness of the great ball and his ability to create, and we thereby learned about our own ability to create.

He taught us three important things about creating:

1. The journey to the goal is no less important than reaching the goal.

2. The thoughts you are engaged in during creation are the ones that affect the result.

3. Nothing stands in the way of will.

We were connected to both the physical world and the higher worlds. That is, even if we drank water, we also drank light. Even if we ate food grown on the earth, we always had barrels of light at our home and ate from them. We always coated the earth with brown light energy. When we created homes, we always coated them with white light energy. The light was an inseparable part of our lives, and alongside life here we saw, felt, ate, drank, and breathed the light we pulled from the higher worlds.

In the 'early days' era, people's consciousness was different. It was totally clean, and it enabled us to live in peace and in constant connection with ourselves, with the universe, and with the higher worlds. At any given moment, each human being aspired to create without limits, to develop, and to help those around him. Each soul arrived with a certain mission and it made the utmost effort to fulfill this life mission: to develop the thing which would best serve itself and those around it. Human beings who had trouble doing it enlisted the help of others, and harmony and peace were shared by everyone.

I long for my friends, those souls who left this world and went up to the higher worlds long ago. They were great, special souls.

We knew we were not only physical beings, but that everything that existed in this world, including human beings, was energy. And if everything was energy, everything could be changed and moved.

In order for a person to change and move energy, he first needs to know that he possesses the ability to do so. He needs to see the energy, feel it, and at the moment of truth focus on the goal and put it into action. We had fundamental rules that guided us: we were allowed to move and change energy as long as we did not harm another person, did not harm ourselves, and did not harm all that was around us.

Each one of us was happy with what he had, and it was therefore fun living here. There were no comparisons or competition; we had a common goal to keep the divine spark burning. In order to do that, we created, learned, developed, sought each other's help, laughed, sang, and danced. In order to get help from one another, there was no need to ask. Each one of us saw and heard the other and was always willing to help. We worked in stupendous cooperation. We created everything with our own hands, with constant help from the higher worlds.

I have been living in this world for a very long time and I have experienced the turnover of many generations. Yet there has never been a period like the era where we were granted the ability to create life and produce the greatest miracle for the first time since this world's creation—the children.

Yes! This was the most exciting period I have experienced in my life, and truth be told, in the current state of affairs this memory provides me with the happiness and power to go on.

Tomorrow will be a joyful day for all of you. At sundown, you will be experiencing what used to be our daily routine in the 'early days' era. All families are invited."

The oldest of souls ended his message with a request:

"Dear, beloved souls, I am confident that we can eliminate the negativity epidemic if we all return and live the way we used to live in the 'early days' era. I ask you to share what I told you with your families and pray for a return to those days when only positivity existed in this world."

Peace and quiet prevailed and everyone was able to imagine the daily routine of the "early days." Everyone left the meeting content and knew that as long as there was common will and joint prayer, they would be able to recreate the "early days" era. There was a clear hope and a clear target: *a return to the "early days" era.*

The last meeting left its mark in the hearts of the participants. One could feel it in the air; everyone was talking about the "early days" and about the desire to live like in those days. The meeting ended at midday. Throughout the rest of the day, each one spent time with his family. The excitement was incredible, and at night, many were not able to sleep in anticipation for the next day.

The awaited moment arrived. Toward sundown, masses of people gathered, eagerly waiting for the "early days" experience.

At sundown, the gates of the heavens opened and golden light energy started to rain down, bringing happiness into everyone's hearts. A spectacularly beautiful layer of golden colored light was spread. The ceremony of the "early days" experience had begun. Numerous wind instruments cheered on; the sound from the ram's horn sounds purified the energy around them. Their hearts were overcome by the sounds of joy, laughter, and infinite contentment. These were blessed moments for everyone.

Immense quantities of light started to come down from the skies. Light energies of different colors filled this world and were piled up on the streets. Light pools, light dunes, and light waterfalls of different colors took shape. Toys made of light, sand boxes, and slides made of light were created.

Everyone looked around and was stunned by the magnificent scene created before them. The babies and children were running everywhere and enjoying the light. The adults watched with great pleasure.

The oldest of souls faced everyone while standing on a hill and explained:

"This is how we lived every day in the 'early days' era. We enjoyed abundance. We lived and breathed the light and it was a daily, inseparable commodity in our lives. Look how your children enjoy swimming in the light pools that fill them with love and purify them of all the energy accumulated within them. Look at how the ground is covered with light and babies are crawling on it, eating the light and taking pleasure in rolling in it. When they eat light, they eat positive information. All of this can be experienced, not only today, but each day. Let's make a pact; let's aspire to return to these 'early days.'"

He finished speaking and everyone cheered with incredible roars. Everyone was excited, flooded with love and happiness.

When he finished speaking, the oldest of souls stepped off the hill. While stepping down towards the crowd, he stumbled and his foot was injured. He had never experienced such a thing and he saw it as a warning sign. He realized he must go back home and try to understand the meaning of it. While walking with his wife towards their home, they shared with each other the wonderful feeling the event left within them. The oldest of souls even told her that he was so full of love and excitement that he wanted to teach everyone about the "early days." He believed that the more they knew about this era, the more they would want to go back and live as they once had lived.

When they got home, the oldest of soul's wife made tea and put the pitcher on the table.

"Join me, my dear," she invited.

As he rose from his seat, the oldest of souls felt pain in his injured foot.

"There is something I want to share with you," he said after he sat down.

The oldest of souls told her about the pain he felt in his foot and she nodded as if she knew.

Profound silence prevailed in the room. Neither of them spoke. They both knew something was about to happen. Although she already knew, she waited for her beloved husband to discover the message himself.

After a prolonged and soothing silence, the oldest of souls understood that he needed to leave for a long seclusion. He decided that the next day, he would leave at dawn to the forest for an unlimited period, and would return once he felt it was right to do so. The oldest of souls went to sleep and his wife packed for him all that was needed.

The oldest of souls woke up before dawn and set off. He had been serving other people for a long time, and this seclusion was essential for him. On his way to the forest, some thoughts came to his mind, "What is going to happen in this world? Will people really put an effort to go back and live the way we used to live in the 'early days' era? The great ball took the suffering from their children. Now, when they do not suffer, will they be willing to renounce their past habits, to change things within themselves? And if so, I need to teach them all that I know."

The oldest of souls settled in the forest and went into a deep inner observation. When he closed his eyes, he saw black clouds approaching him, settling before him, and then disappearing. The vision repeated five times. The fifth time, he tried to understand the meaning of the vision.

"What does this symbolize to me?" he asked.

The answer was not late in coming. The great ball was revealed in front of his eyes and spoke to him:

"My dear son, it is time for you to return to me. Your time in this world has ended. In four moons and seven days you will return to live in the higher worlds, close to me and to your brothers whom you miss so much."

A smile spread over the oldest of souls' face. He had been waiting for the day when he would be allowed to leave this world and return to his source, and the thought filled him with tranquility and serenity. At the same time, he started getting worried about life in this world. He could not figure out why the great ball chose specifically then to do it, therefore he turned to the great ball:

"My dear father, why now? Why, when all people want to make a change in their lives, do you want me to leave them? If I do not lead them and do not help them, who will do it?"

"My dear son," answered the great ball, "I sent you away from them in order to see if they really want to make a change in their lives. A real change starts from within, when someone decides to make it. It does not depend on anything external. They know what negative is and what positive is, and they will need to choose what they want in their lives. While people make their choices in their lives, I ask that during the next four moons you recall your life in this world and prepare yourself to return to your source."

"If they choose to go with the positive, will you let me stay with them?" asked the oldest of souls.

The great ball laughed with love and replied, "For this, too, I have a plan."

From this moment, the oldest of souls dedicated the time he had left in this world to deep observation of his life in this world. Each day he would start the observation at dawn and finish at sunset. He observed his whole life, collected memories, difficulties, contemplations, and mainly observed how the knowledge from the "early days" era served both him and others, during various life situations and periods.

As days went by, people went back to their life routines and the "early days" experience dissipated. It was hard for them to change and let go of all the habits that were ingrained in them. Some of them wanted help; others wanted someone else to do the job for them. Delegates of the families came to seek help from the oldest of souls, but once they understood that he had gone for an unknown period of seclusion, some were driven to despair, others to doubt. A new seed was created in their consciousness: "Only the oldest of souls can! Only he can use the knowledge from the 'early days.' We cannot. He came from there; he has something special we don't have."

Once the oldest of soul's wife heard about the doubt, she felt obligated to help.

Since the time the great ball decided people would take part in the creation of man, she found herself involved with childbirth. She was fortunate to have been the first midwife. The great miracle happened every day in front of her eyes. Day by day she was fortunate to touch the purity of life, the little, helpless babies, full of strength and power, being emitted from their mother's womb.

She had great influence on women, therefore she decided to have a gathering at her house with the women she was closest to, and help them in any way she could.

"Two days ago, I was present for the birth of Hope," she shared with them. "When Hope came out of her mother's womb and took her first breath, I broke into tears. This time, it was not out of burning excitement inside me, but out of sadness. I held her as close as I could, breathed her sweet scent and thought 'What would happen with all the babies if people did not choose the positive?' Hope felt my concern and shared with me her most intimate feelings. She explained to me telepathically that she was very happy to come to this world. She explained that she was given a chance to contribute to our world by helping to cleanse many souls. Hope told me she was a soul who had waited a very long time to come down to this world. She said she had many tasks to perform and was grateful for the great privilege given to her. She also shared with me that she already knew about the negativity in our world and its implications on everyone. Lastly, she told me she also knew that the oldest of souls might need to leave this world soon."

"I wondered what she meant, and she replied: 'The great ball understood that in order for people to perform a real internal change, he must send the oldest of souls away from them. A real change starts from within. The person chooses it, wants it, and never gives it up. True will does not depend on any external cause.'"

"l thanked her for the information she shared with me and gave her back to her mother."

"After Hope's birth, I returned home and performed a deep observation on the conversation I had had with her. I felt yearning for my husband and wanted him to return home. Now, in my heart, I know he will return home, but if people do not uproot the doubt they have embedded in their consciousness, he will return to the higher worlds. I ask each and every one of you to release love from your heart; give it to your spouses and to every family you know. Explain to them the situation and recruit them to make the change we hope for."

Four moons passed and the oldest of souls finished his mission. He observed himself and called for the great ball.

"Dear father, I have completed my mission. What should I do now? What is the situation in this world?"

The great ball responded, "Most people went back to live their lives as usual. They have decided they cannot change themselves. They have decided that you have something they do not have: special abilities that only the ones who used to live in the 'early days' era have."

"I do not understand," cried the oldest of souls, "Why do they do it to themselves? We are all built the same; we all have the extraordinary divine spark and the same abilities. They have each other and they have you. What more could they need?"

The great ball replied:

"The easiest and most convenient thing for human beings to do is simply to say 'I cannot do it.'"

"I still do not understand," the oldest of souls retorted. "After all, they know that if they return to the path they chose in the past, their children will suffer."

"Sadly, human beings forget quickly," Said the great ball. "In the past, I could not see my children suffer and their parents tormented, therefore I came down to this world, froze it with great light and with a twinkling of an eye took the suffering from the children. During your long life in this world, you have realized that every time I have intervened and helped them without them taking an active part, the reality I created did not last long, and they went back to their old bad habits.

My beloved son, the children are a joint creation of their parents and me. Their lives are greatly affected by their parents, and this is why they will live in this world according to the way their ancestors and their parent lived.

If parents want their children to live in health and happiness and fulfill the destiny of their soul in this world, they must take full responsibility of their own lives and change themselves; they have to uproot the negativity from their lives and stay connected to their inner selves and to the higher worlds. I am always there for them, to help them fulfill whatever they wish for, but they have to want it and do more on their own. And you, my beloved son, I ask you to return home, talk with your wife about everything you went through, and make your farewells."

The oldest of souls recalled all the suffering that existed among human beings and the thought that he would leave them like that and return to the higher worlds weighed upon his heart. "Father, please leave me here just a little longer and I will make them understand that they can live the way we used to live in the 'early days' era," he begged.

"Having you stay will not help," replied the great ball. "You cannot force them to change. They will need to find out that in order to live in this world in health and in peace, and in order to fulfill their soul's purpose, they must use the natural abilities I planted within them. Each one of them has inner listening abilities, inner visual abilities, abilities that enable communicating without words, abilities to be connected to oneself and to the higher worlds and get answers from within. They will need to choose to use them. The moment they realized you are from the 'early days' era, they started believing that only you can use the abilities everyone used back then."

The great ball added, "As time goes by, they will grow apart from themselves, they will suffer more, and will believe less and less that they have these abilities. This is why your task has ended. Had you been an ordinary person, one who leads a normal life and experiences suffering, you would have been able to lead the people to the change we hope for.

Had you been a simple and average person who deals with what the others deal with in their everyday lives, you would have been able to show them that they can use these natural abilities and maintain their health as you do. However, this is not the situation. Your blessed life had no suffering thanks to your constant use of the natural abilities that are planted in every human being. You have contributed so much to this world and the time has now come for you to return to me."

The oldest of souls turned to the great ball and thanked him for all the years in which the great ball served as a father to him. The great ball got inside him and gave him a loving, fatherly hug.

"I am happy to come back to you, I miss the kingdom of heaven," announced the oldest of souls.

"Go back to your home, my dear son, and bid farewell to your wife and to this world," ended the great ball.

On that day, the oldest of souls started the journey back to his home. He shared with his wife everything he had experienced and all that was about to happen. His wife shared with him everything that had happened while he was away.

They hugged and tears of acceptance shed from their eyes. The oldest of souls had three days left in this world. He chose to stay home with his wife. After two days, the oldest of souls returned to the forest for another day of seclusion, and since then no one has seen him.

Part B

A New Beginning

Chapter 7

A New Beginning

Thousands of years have passed since then, along with many generations. Man's consciousness and inner needs have completely changed, causing this world to completely change.

The intensity and complexity of human life has greatly increased. Countless new and amazing developments have been made in science, technology, healing arts, medicine, and so much more. On the other hand, this added complexity has brought with it a fog that pervades human life. It clouds our understanding, making it difficult to see good from bad, right from wrong, and moral from immoral. People have moved away from one another, from their family cell, from nature, from the Creator, and especially from their inner selves.

The world has witnessed a cruel reality in which people experience in their everyday lives pain, fear, sorrow, war, uncertainty, and more. People experience suffering in different ways and at different ages.

I, too, have encountered suffering in my life. The first time was when I was a baby. My father passed away when I was eight months old, without any warning. This was unbearable for my mother. She was angry with both my father, may he rest in peace, and with the Creator for leaving her alone so young, helpless and hurt, with three little children.

Life in this world went on. I grew up, and from the outside, everything was fine. When I was two years old, my mother remarried, and thus two families were united into one. Suddenly, my life changed. In just one day, I had a new father and three new siblings.

My parents dedicated their life to us. My mother was there for us every moment of our lives, but the painful loss at such an early age and the circumstances of her life did not allow her to give me her healing love. My entire life I saw in her eyes the sorrow and pain she carried with her. My heart was sensitive towards her; I felt her pain inside me but I never asked about my father or showed any sadness.

Early in my life, I felt emptiness inside me. I wanted so much to hear my father, see him, and hug him, even just once. I felt that in order to live, I must fill this emptiness and I thus found an escape. Every day, I withdrew into myself; I would meet my father and the Creator, and would fill myself with love, confidence and inner peace. I would talk with them about myself, about my family, and about the world. I would ask questions and receive answers. Every day I would go about my life and see the world from the eyes of a child who is connected to her inner self and the universe. There was a huge gap between the everyday life I lived in the external world and the inner life I experienced with the Creator and with my father.

My connection with my father and with the Creator was so strong, that I would not go anywhere without them present. As a child, I walked in the world with joy, a self-existential security, and a strong connection to my inner self and to the higher worlds.

At a young age, I chose to heal people. I studied classical homeopathy and practiced homeopathy for seven years. Early on, I understood that I could not bear children's suffering, and more than that, it was hard for me to hear all the horror stories, the fear and helplessness parents experienced while their children suffered. With the knowledge that I had, I did all I could to help them. But already then *something inside me would not let me accept the common reality* that the solution to the children's suffering exists only in doctors and therapists. I knew there was something else, something we do not understand, something that was missing and that I had to find.

I then brought my first child to the world. My self-existential security dismantled on the very same day. Fear entered and controlled my life. I was afraid that something would happen to my child; since my father passed away without any warning, it could happen to anyone.

My first child opened my past wounds and enabled me to go through a process of deep reconnection to my inner self. I wanted with all my heart to understand why children suffer in the world and how their suffering could be uprooted. The burning desire to prevent suffering from happening to my son and the inner drive to reveal the solution that would save all children did not leave me even for a moment. I went on living the way I did in my childhood: on the outside I led a normal life; inside, I was secluded and listened deeply to myself, to my father, and to the Creator, knowing that only from this place the answer would come.

I observed my relationship with my son and started to see my influence on his life. As time went by, the fog lifted and the picture became definite and clear.

My son gave me the greatest gift of all. He showed me the direct effect I have on him. I found out there was a direct relation between his physical and emotional suffering and my emotional-mental situation, without exception. Everything passed to him without words. The more I was balanced, the more he was balanced and did not suffer.

I continued to heal people and observed the relationships between parents and children. I saw the connection between the suffering of the children and their parents' emotional-mental state. I noticed that when I gave the parents, as part of their children's healing process, guidance that led them to change things in themselves, there was acceleration in the children's healing. With time, there was a significant improvement in their health. The children got sick less often, and if they got sick, their healing process was fast.

The picture became clear. *The solution to children's suffering lies in their parents*. There is a connection between children's suffering and their parents, therefore in order to prevent suffering and to heal the children, it is not enough to send them to the best doctors or therapists. Parents need to take part in their children's healing process.

I saw before my eyes the power of parents: they are an immense force, having tremendous influence and natural innate abilities. Yet this powerful force does not know it can play an immense role in healing. I saw strong hands that can change any life reality but they are tied and unaware of their great power.

I wanted to uproot the helplessness and paralyzing fear that exists in parents when they see their child suffer, to awaken the natural healing power that exists within them so they could call upon this power in love, in determination, and in valor, for the sake of their children.

I wanted with all my heart to grant parents in general and mothers in particular the best gift they could ask for, which is the ability to prevent suffering in their children and help them in any state of suffering.

I then went on a new journey in which I asked new questions and looked passionately for the answers. *I wanted to find the path that would lead parents to take part in healing themselves and their children.* I understood that it had to be simple, clear, accessible, and easy to learn; a way that every person could successfully use in his everyday life in order to take part in healing himself and his children.

In the new journey, I understood that the abilities I used in my childhood so naturally in order to cope with my own suffering—the immense emptiness that was inside me—are natural and innate abilities to every human being. These are inner listening abilities, inner visual abilities, telepathic abilities that enable every human being to communicate without words, and abilities to connect to his inner self and to the higher worlds and get answers from within.

I started to use these abilities in healing those seeking help and there was a tremendous breakthrough; I discovered that I was able to see the source of people's suffering and uproot it from their lives. While closing my eyes, I observed the energetic body of those seeking help and saw what they had experienced in the past. I understood the relation between what they experienced in the past and their emotional, mental, and physical suffering. I also understood that in order to heal them, I needed to correct the past experience I saw and take it out of their body.

Generally, throughout my experience in healing people of all ages and in various suffering situations, from common issues to life threatening ones, I have seen the influence parents have on their children's lives. But the breakthrough I had has enabled me to see that influence on a deeper level. I discovered that the passage of energy from parents to children is a natural process and is beyond our control. *I saw how parents' past experiences pass to their children.* These past experiences reside in the child's energetic body as if they belonged to him, influencing his health. Moreover, *I witnessed that when I correct and cleanse the past experience from the parent, there is significant alleviation, acceleration of the healing process, and even complete recovery of the child.*

I have continued using these abilities for years in healing thousands of cases and performed deep observations on people and on parent-child relationships. After years of persistence without compromise and a burning desire to prevent suffering and uproot it from the lives of children, I have discovered knowledge that I named "*Healing Parents.*"

The "Healing Parents" knowledge is my gift to every person, and to parents in particular, so they can take an active part in healing themselves and their children as well as prevent suffering. As years went by, I discovered more parts of the knowledge, used it, developed it, and made it simple, clear, practical, and suitable to our lifetime and to every person.

Many questions might be popping into your head now: "What am I to do? How can I change? What should I change? How will these changes influence my children? How am I at all related to my children's suffering? How come I can heal?"

It is important that you understand that the solution to your children's suffering lies in your hands. Turning into a healing parent is a process. *The first step in being a healing parent is to understand that you affect your children physically, emotionally, and mentally, and to take full responsibility for your life—to focus on what you can correct and improve in yourself.*

Stop here and read the last paragraph again. It is important that you internalize the message I give you. This internalization will enable you to take an active part in healing your children by correcting yourself, and as a result stop the development of suffering and prevent it in yourself and your children.

Later on, you will be able to take part in your children's healing by using more of the *"Healing Parents"* knowledge to directly alleviate their suffering and heal them.

Some of you and your loved ones suffer more than others do. I am sorry for all your suffering and wish I could take it away from you in an instant, but I cannot. Every day I encounter cases of suffering and try with all my might to remove it. The suffering is huge and I alone cannot help all of humanity. The solution to suffering lies within the parents. Only when parents take the reins, when they understand that they are the best healers for their children and take an active part in healing themselves and their children, can we succeed in uprooting suffering from humanity.

People have moved away from their inner selves and from the higher worlds, but their love towards their children has remained. A burning desire lies within them, moving them to give, listen, and act for their children without limits.

The necessary change in the world can be made only thanks to your power of love. When people go through a process in which they reconnect to their inner selves; their heart will open and they will be capable of releasing healing love to their loved ones and the ones surrounding them. People will understand their role in the world, observe what they need to correct in themselves, and realize how much they are needed and how much influence they have. They will therefore choose to take an active and positive part in everything in which they are involved. People will be united and will act together for the realization of one goal: *releasing the children to complete freedom.*

From the next chapter on, I will reveal to you techniques that can help you stop the development of suffering and prevent it in yourself and your children.

Part C

~~

The Power Within Us

Chapter 8

The Life Center of the Person

The great ball created children who were like him. As long as they were living with him in the higher worlds, they were made—just like him—of light, but before he gave them freedom and sent them down to this world, he changed their form.

He created the human body so that it comprises three bodies: a physical body, a mental body (consciousness), and an energetic body. He took his children, the sparks of light, and inserted them into the energetic body. *The spark of light is the soul of the human being.* When a human being arrives in this world, his energetic body contains the soul, which holds the divine spark. The divine spark is exactly as it was on the day of its creation. The divine spark has all the qualities of the great ball.

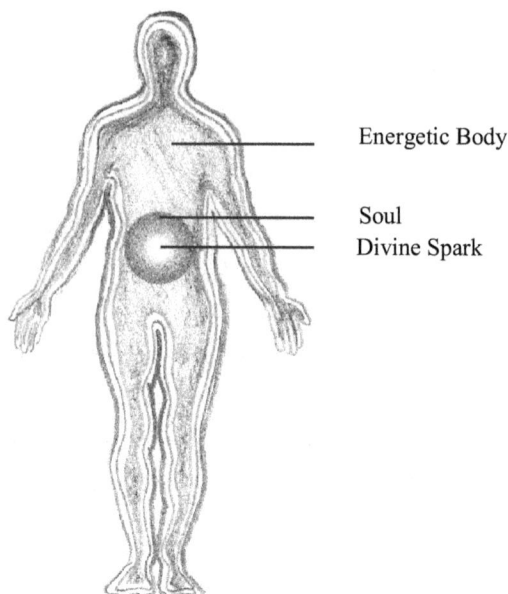

Illustration 1: The energetic body contains the soul, which holds the divine spark

Harm done to any one of the bodies causes suffering. Suffering is any situation that hinders a person's normal function, whether it can be diagnosed by the five senses or by laboratory tests, or whether it cannot be explained, diagnosed or labeled with a name of a "disease."

Let's learn what each body includes, how it can be harmed, and what its role is:

The Physical Body

The physical body that the great ball created includes all of the body's systems: the body organs, skeleton, tissues, bodily fluids, and so on. The emotional system is included in this body as well.

Harming the Physical Body

Harm done to the physical body will be manifested as harm to the body's various systems, to the skeleton, to the tissues, etc. These injuries will take the form of high blood pressure, spinal problems, laryngitis, and many other physical injuries people suffer from.

Harm done to the emotional system will take the form of extreme mood swings, anxiety, panic attacks, acute timidity, addictions, etc.

The Mental Body (Consciousness)

The great ball placed consciousness in the mental body. In it reside thoughts, thinking patterns, and conditioning ("if… then…").

Harming the Mental Body

Harm done to the mental body will be manifested as diminished cerebral capacity, for example: forgetfulness, attention deficit disorders, senility, constant troublesome thoughts, obsessive thoughts, suicidal thoughts, and so on.

The Roles of the Physical and Mental Bodies

The physical and mental bodies serve as bodyguards for the energetic body. They constitute a wall of defense against breaches of the energetic body. They do this by warding off any external element that tries to penetrate them and any internal element that interrupts them, thus preventing penetration to the energetic body and harm to the divine spark. In this manner, they serve the energetic body best and allow the divine spark to burn in full force.

The Energetic Body

This body cannot be perceived with our five senses. However, it affects our lives tremendously. There, you can find the source of suffering, therefore performing work on this body is the key to preventing and healing suffering.

The Role of the Energetic Body

The energetic body preserves the soul and the divine spark within it by serving as a wall that blocks energetic memories from getting into the soul. It also supplies vital force—fire—to the mental and physical body.

The Divine Spark

The divine spark is the DNA of the great ball, and it exists in all of us. It is the seed, the heredity of the great ball. It is the divine part that exists in each and every one of us.

The divine spark holds all of the Creator's abilities. By using the divine spark, the person gets freedom: freedom of health, economic freedom, freedom to express feelings, freedom to choose an occupation, freedom to control his life, freedom to set the course of his life, freedom to be everywhere at the same time, to experience love, joy, hope, courage, compassion, patience, acceptance, passion, vigor, and to create without limits.

The Divine Spark's Role

The supreme role of the divine spark is to remain burning, thus allowing the person it inhabits to make the most of the Creator's abilities. The divine spark does so by giving life to all three bodies. *It is the center of the person's life*, it is the engine of the human machine, and so the brighter it burns, the healthier the person. The divine spark lends the three bodies its power, allowing them to perform their roles in the best way possible and to protect the person.

The divine spark can be likened to fire, while the energetic body can be likened to a bonfire: the greater the flame in the divine spark, the greater the bonfire in the energetic body. The brighter the divine spark burns, the brighter the energetic body burns. When the energetic body burns brightly, it gives the physical body and mental body powerful life force to remove any element that invades them.

The best situation for the divine spark is when all three bodies are healthy; that is, working harmoniously and free of all suffering. This harmonious state allows the divine spark to burn brightly and freely, which enables the person it inhabits to realize his full potential.

The divine spark may burn at various degrees. As long as combustion exists, even the slightest bit, the spark burns and the person is alive in this world.

The more you invest in lighting a fire, the bigger the bonfire burns. To preserve the fire, you must always be vigilant and you must keep working. You have to feed the fire with more wood, twigs, sticks, and other kindling, or it will fade—and, with time, die. It is the same with the divine spark. The more you care for it, work with it, and use it, the stronger it gets. *The more people use the qualities that are in the divine spark, i.e. the ability to create, rejoice, influence, accept, and so forth, the more their divine spark burns.*

The energetic body uses the divine spark's fire for our everyday life. The energetic body provides the person fire—vital force—with which the person acts. The greater the burning of the divine spark, the greater the vital force of the person, and thus the healthier the person.

In their everyday lives, people unconsciously hurt their inner flame, their vital force, and as a result suffer. In order to distance suffering from your life, it is important for me to share with you how people harm their inner fire, their vital force, and what you can do in order to prevent this in your life and the life of your loved ones.

What Causes Harm to a Person's Energetic Body?

There are two paths that may lead to harm in the energetic body: an active way and a passive way.

The Passive Way

In the passive way, people take no stand and fail to do anything to extinguish the fire or to keep it burning. They just stand in place and do nothing with the fire, until the bonfire fades on its own.

These people do nothing to develop and advance in their lives. They make no effort and assume no responsibility; they do not leave their comfort zone, but they do not harm others either. They stay on the same course for years. In some cases, these are either people who "bury their head in the sand" and do not see what is going on in their lives or people who would rather live in denial than deal with reality.

The Active Way

In the active way, you do something to extinguish the fire. You can, for example, pour water on it, throw sand on it, take out all the firewood, and give it to others, so your fire dies off. You can smother the fire at once using one big tarp; you can call for outside help, or ask your neighbors to come help you extinguish your fire.

In the active way, two paths lead to harming the energetic body:

The first path is powerful penetration into the physical and/or mental body, in a way that prevents these two bodies from blocking the entry into the energetic body.

The second path is through weak, repetitive penetration into the physical and/or mental bodies. Despite the penetration being weak, it has a *cumulative effect* on the energetic body.

In the following passage, I will describe in detail the two paths.

1. Powerful Penetration to the Physical and/or Mental Body

Powerful penetration into the physical and/or mental body may be caused by any sudden, forceful event that affects a person's life in a negative way. For example, a car accident, sexual assault, childbirth, miscarriage, emotional abuse, bad news, attempted suicide, or violent bacteria attacking a weak body. The event is so powerful that the physical and mental bodies are unable to deal with it, and it enters the energetic body directly and embeds itself into the soul. In such cases, the event is registered as an energetic memory and the divine spark, the source of the fire, is harmed.

An *energetic memory* is any negative experience the person had, which was so forceful that it left its mark on the soul or the energetic body as an unforgettable memory.

Energetic memories take up space in the person's soul. The more energetic memories there are, the more congested the soul becomes, and the memories "squeeze" the divine spark within it, like stones that are thrown onto a bonfire and cause the flame to fade.

At best, the stone is a little one, with little effect on the fire, but sometimes there are many stones or huge boulders that threaten to "choke" the fire. *The reason the energetic body fails to ward off the energy that comes in* is that in order to deal with the energy—the experience—that penetrated, it needs to give all its fire all at once, and this might risk the person's life. Therefore, the person's denial mechanism exists. The person cannot deal at that time with incoming information and therefore it is buried in the soul. In cases like these, the soul—which holds the higher wisdom—awaits until it sees that the energetic body has enough vital force to give the person, and that the person is capable of dealing with the buried experience. At the right moment, the soul will release the energy into the energetic body, and it will relay it to the other two bodies as suffering. The experience may remain in the soul for years and one day erupt as suffering.

One of our purposes in this world is to extract from the soul all of the "stones" that were thrown into it; that is, to cleanse the soul, to extract all the energetic memories, thus allowing the divine spark to burn intensely.

There are extreme cases in which powerful penetration into one of the bodies leads to a situation in which the intrusive element takes over that body. The energetic body is required to give up all of its fire, its strength, all at once, in order to save the injured body. *In these cases, the denial mechanism does not work*, and the energetic body immediately provides a large amount of life force, or fire, to the other two bodies. In such cases, the fire within the energetic body dwindles in a way that is life threatening, as the fire may be extinguished. Examples of this are illness due to violent bacteria, extreme panic, financial ruin, or bad news that may cause a heart attack or another life-threatening situation. The reason *the energetic body cannot hold back the entering energy* is that it is weak; it does not have enough vital force to share.

When you use the *"Healing Parents"* knowledge for healing, you perform an observation and work on the person's energetic body. During this type of observation, you see energies that are located in the energetic body and cause the person to suffer. Energies in the energetic body take shape. It is possible to see the energy as objects of any type, and as past experiences the person had. The energy seen in the energetic body is energetic memory. It is kept in the person's body and is the reason for his suffering. When the energy trapped in the energetic body is removed, the person is released from his suffering.

The following is an example of powerful penetration to the physical body or the mental body, where the bodies cannot ward off the penetration. The energy enters the energetic body and sits in the soul as an energetic memory:

A 35-year-old man sought treatment due to chest pains. The pain he was experiencing was like knife stabbings. My observation of his energetic body revealed to me a memory that dated years back. In his energetic body, I saw in the chest area an anchor-shaped piece of iron as well as a great amount of water and I extracted them. All of a sudden, I saw a four-year-old boy sitting there, crying. I approached him and struck up a telepathic conversation:

"What are you doing here, sweetie?"

- "I'm looking for my mommy."

"Where is your mother?"

- "I don't know."

I removed the child from the energetic body. I continued my observation and saw wooden planks that looked like a ship's deck, and other objects that looked like parts of a ship. I extracted all of them from the man's energetic body.

When I completed the healing work, I asked the man what the memory meant. He told me that when he was four-and-a-half years old, his mother fell ill and had to leave him for two months, after which he no longer accepted her. The ship motif that kept repeating itself inside his body had to do with his father, who was a sailor.

In this case, the person experienced in his childhood an emotional experience that was intolerable. At that point, he could not cope with the experience so he repressed it and it entered directly into his energetic body and settled in his soul. That childhood experience is like a stone sitting inside the soul and causes the fire of the divine spark to fade.

Removing energetic memories from the soul creates space for the divine spark and enables it to exist, to burn intensely again. When this man got to an age in which he could cope with the experience, the soul—which has the supreme wisdom—released the experience that had settled in it to his energetic body. The energetic body released the experience as suffering in his physical body, in this case chest pains. The man in fact was put face to face with the past through suffering. This is the soul's way of enabling the person to cleanse the accumulated energy due to the past experience. In the example above, until the man felt pain, he did not know there was something inside him that was taking some of his vital force, his fire.

The suffering of the physical body and the mental body is liberated in the exact locations where the work on the energetic body is performed. In the previous example, the work focused on the chest of the energetic body. Thus, the same area in the physical body was rendered free from pain. After four sessions and the help of the patient's daily work, his heart was freed from the suffering caused by that past experience. The memory that inhabited his mental body, his consciousness, changed; he can now look at the world through different glasses.

To sum up: In this example, the person had experienced a childhood trauma that he could not deal with. The experience entered his energetic body directly and imprinted as an energetic memory in the soul. Years later, when he had the ability to deal with that experience, the memory embedded into his soul transferred to the energetic body and manifested as suffering in the other two bodies. Thus, this person had the chance to cleanse his soul from the past's memory and enable his divine spark to burn again.

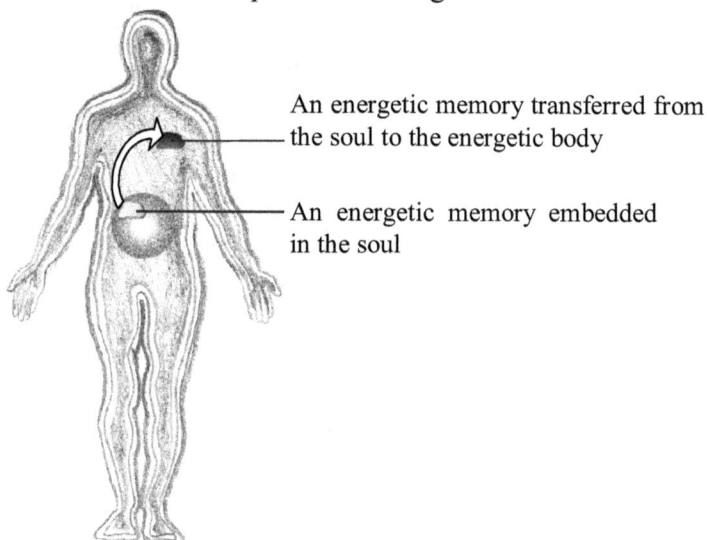

An energetic memory transferred from the soul to the energetic body

An energetic memory embedded in the soul

Illustration 2: release of energetic memory from the soul

People go through negative experiences during their lives from the moment of conception, thus their energetic body and their soul get stained with energetic memories that influence their health condition and their life in general.

One of the soul's ways to cleanse itself is through suffering. The soul releases negative energy—a negative past experience—that has been buried inside it through suffering, thus bringing the person face to face with the past experience. The person sees and feels the suffering, and not the cause for the suffering, which is a past experience. As a result, he wants to get rid of the symptoms and not the true cause.

If you or your loved ones currently experience suffering, accept the suffering as positive and understand that it serves the cleansing and purification of the soul. When people suffer, especially when helpless children are involved, I know it is extremely hard to grasp and to accept their suffering. However, when a person accepts the suffering, he enables his body to concentrate his energies on healing. He is available to focus on the essence, on all that needs to be healed, and on the things that will contribute to the healing process.

2. Weak, Repetitive Penetration into the Physical Body and/or Mental Body

So far, I have shared with you how the energetic body is hurt as a result of powerful penetration to the physical and/or mental bodies. Now I will share with you how the energetic body gets hurt due to weak, repetitive penetration into the physical body and/or mental body.

This type of harm in the energetic body, in the bonfire, is made by various elements people produce themselves. *In this active way, people behave in a way that hurts themselves and others, either consciously or not. The harm is caused by any negative intention, thought, or deed they perform toward themselves, others, or their environment.*

Harmful elements that people produce penetrate to the physical and mental bodies. The energetic body lends its life force, its fire, in order to ward off the harming element. It does so consistently and persistently, but if the harming elements continue to "pound" constantly, daily, the energetic body weakens.

In this situation, the energetic body "wastes" some of its fire on warding off the harming elements. The fire within the energetic body fades, until the energetic body no longer possesses the life force it once had. It has only a little life force left to give to the other two bodies in order to ward off harming elements. The result is that hostile elements can easily penetrate, inhabit it, and harm the divine spark. Moreover, in this situation the person does not use the fire for self-fulfillment and growth but for survival.

The harmful elements can be at different risk levels: those that are life threatening and those that are not. The intrusive elements might be external or internal.

An *External Causing Element* is either something the person does, or something that enters a person from the outside. This includes food that can harm the body, medicine, gossip, lies, arguments, anger, cursing, hatred from another person, alcohol, tobacco, drugs, sex addiction, and emotional or physical abuse.

An *Internal Causing Element* is everything that the person experiences within himself. For example, not keeping one's word, deceit, unrelenting feelings of guilt, obsessive thoughts, self hatred, worry, fears, jealousy, anger, grudges, suicidal thoughts, and one of the most powerful pathogens of modern times—repression:

> *The repression of thoughts*
>
> *The repression of emotions*
>
> *The repression of desires, and*
>
> *The repression of illness*

Repression is a daily occurrence in modern society, and in most cases, we do not even notice it. It appears to be the normal reality in which we live.

Repression is a situation whereby something physical or emotional is trying to surface, but the person chooses to keep it inside; or alternately, something has surfaced and the person wants to force it back inside. Physical repression is, for instance, a migraine that is being treated by designated pain relief medicine. A migraine is an external expression of internal energy that has accumulated in the head area. In order to heal the migraine, the internal cause—the accumulated energy—should be removed. The disappearance of the migraine as a result of consuming the medicine is repression and not healing. Emotional repression, for example, is feelings of anger that a person chooses not to express, or desires a person relinquishes.

The burning intensity of the spark within you and your children also depends on the way you choose to handle your suffering. Remember that one of the most powerful pathogens of modern life is *repression* of thoughts, emotions, desires, and illness. The way suffering is treated has great significance, and I wish to elaborate on it.

When a person is suffering from a problem, it is important to treat him as a whole, rather than just treating the specific problem. This type of perspective is called a *holistic approach.* For instance, when a person suffers from an eye infection, a holistic approach will treat the suffering person as a whole, rather than only the eye. We want to find *the cause* for his suffering and *remove it.* We do not want to simply get rid of the symptom, such as the eye infection in the above example, but rather the cause. Examples of the causes of suffering are frustration, worry, stress, fear, a broken heart, a traumatic experience such as a car accident, a difficult childbirth, and so on. Treating the cause will eliminate the suffering.

Contrary to this holistic approach, which treats the causes rather than just the physical, mental, and emotional effects, conventional medicine typically focuses on removing symptoms. Conventional medicine tries to get rid of the suffering in every possible way, and if needed, by exercising great external force. This is a process of *repression* and it leads to the energetic body's weakening. The energetic body has exerted its life force, its fire, in producing suffering, and now it also has to deal with the external elements entering the body.

In many cases, the repression is so intense that the goal is achieved and the suffering is gone. However, the relief is short-lived because *the cause still remains inside*. The energetic body senses the internal cause and acts again. At best, the energetic body will produce the same type of suffering again; but if the repression is too forceful, and the fire in the divine spark is too weak, the energetic body will no longer be able to manifest the same type of suffering, and will use more vital bodily systems to produce a new type of suffering.

When the energetic body burns brightly, it provides the physical body and mental body with a powerful life force to ward off any external or internal causing element that invades them, thus fulfilling its role in preserving the divine spark. A strong energetic body leads the person to a fast recovery, without complications.

Let's take, for example, inflammation in the body: when the physical body is inflamed and the energetic body burns powerfully, a person's immune system will work intensely and drive the body temperature up. The more powerful the fire in the energetic body, the higher the fever, to an extent that does not risk the person's life and will help him heal from the inflammation. The body's ability to raise its temperature indicates a person's high health level. A good example of this can be seen in infants and children: in order to fight an intrusive harming cause, the body quickly raises its temperature to a level that does not constitute risk, and brings them to a quick recovery.

In any situation in which there is injury to the energetic body, the person is preoccupied with "surviving" and cannot use his internal fire for positive purposes that contribute to him as well as to others. Therefore, it is important that you know what you do to yourself as well as what you do to others that harms the burning of your divine spark, your vital force. You also need to know *what you have to do in order to preserve the burning in your divine spark and even to intensify it, thus preventing much suffering.*

You can examine this in the following observation exercise "Preserving the divine spark." This exercise takes five days. It is essential that you perform it. While you are observing, continue reading on in the book.

✍ *Observation Exercise: "Preserving the Divine Spark"*

This exercise requires a pen, a notebook, and an index card.

Close your eyes and allocate five minutes to each of the following sections:

1. Make a list of the things you do that harm your divine spark, your inner fire, your vital force. For example: become angry, worry, take medication, repress feelings, and have bad nutrition or drinking habits.

2. Make a list of at least five things you can do in your everyday life that will intensify the burn in your divine spark, things that will fill you, empower and gladden you. If, for example, drawing makes you feel good, once you draw you intensify the burn in your divine spark. Most people know what is good for them, but they usually, for different reasons, delay doing it for the day after.

3. Let sections (1) and (2) sit with you for five days. Observe your life. Find out how you harm your fire and how you can kindle it. Add to the list as needed.

4. After five days, observe the lists. Choose from each list three things you commit to change or add to your life. Write on a card in one column the

three things that harm your divine spark, and in another column the three things that will intensify the burning in your divine spark. Start performing these things and ignore all the inner conversations, such as "I do not have any power," "I do not have any money," and so on. Just act!

5. Read the card once a day, and read with intent[3]. It will remind you what you do, or should not do, in order to preserve and kindle the fire in your divine spark.

~

CCH Techniques

In the chapter "A New Beginning," I shared with you the breakthrough in which I discovered I could see the source of people's suffering and uproot it from their lives. I saw how past experiences affected their health and I understood that in order to heal the ones seeking help I needed to correct these experiences and remove them.

I performed the correction by changing the way people perceived the experience in the past and the way they coped with it. This way, I changed their

---

[3] See "Reading With Intention" in exercise "Taking Out the Negativity" on page 68.

consciousness from negative to positive. The treatment did not end with correction but with a completion process: I understood that I needed to take out of the energetic body the past experiences I had seen in it— the negative energy accumulated within it—and fill it with positive energies, such as love, happiness, hope, and light energies.

In order to heal, the formula became consistent and clear: correction and completion. This combination led to significant alleviation in suffering, acceleration in the healing process, and to complete healing.

After years of treating this way, I used my therapeutic experience to develop an energetic way of healing, *whose purpose is to prevent suffering and to heal*. It is an energetic way every person can use for himself and his children, without prior experience. The name I have given to this energetic way is *"Completion and Correction Healing,"* or *CCH*. *CCH* includes many energetic tools and techniques by which the completion and correction is performed. Through *CCH, we perform work on the energetic body and influence also the physical body and the mental body*.

As I have mentioned, in order to make a real change in suffering and health situations, we need to work in the energetic world. A real change will take place only by taking out the source of suffering—which is always an accumulation of energy—not by just giving external relief to the suffering person. Providing only external relief might be followed later on by a burst of suffering in various ways.

One of the ways to take out the source of suffering is by using the *CCH Light Technique*.

CCH Light Technique

In the "early days," all human beings were connected to the higher worlds and enjoyed its abundant positive energies, such as love, happiness, and light energies. Using these positive energies kept the soul and the energetic body purified, thus maintaining a powerful and constant burning in their divine spark.

The more people have moved away from their inner selves and from the higher worlds, the less they have used these positive energies. This reality has led to an accumulation of negative energy in the soul and in the energetic body, thus weakening the burning of the divine spark and causing physical, emotional, or mental suffering.

The light is food for the soul and the divine spark. Using *CCH Light Technique,* you will feed the soul and the divine spark with light, and they will thus burn more intensely. In addition, by using *CCH Light Technique*, you can cleanse the energetic body from negative energies that lie within it and cause suffering, allowing you to heal yourself and your loved ones.

Performing *CCH Light Technique*

Light is a positive energy that exists in the higher worlds abundantly. The energy of light is accessible to everyone. I use light every day; using it, I alleviate the suffering of those who seek help, and I am able to heal and empower them. I use the energies of light of different colors and different textures, such as gas, liquid, mud, ointment, lotion, soil, and more.

In fact, everything that exists in this world has an energetic equivalent, made of light energy. You can thus drink it, eat it, use it as a lotion, a blanket, and more. For example, as there is a blanket in the physical world, there is a blanket in the energetic world. So, when you put your children to bed, envision yourself covering them with a white light blanket. The light blanket will protect them and will flow into them light energy throughout the night.

A person who performs CCH Light Technique practices absolute control over his consciousness and unconditional giving. This way he develops inner listening abilities, inner vision abilities, accuracy, and concentration abilities.

You can perform *CCH Light Technique* on yourself as well as on your loved ones. By using *CCH*, every person has the opportunity to take an active part in his own healing process and that of his loved ones.

While performing *CCH Light Technique,* you close your eyes and envision in front of you the person on whom you wish to perform the technique. You pull positive energies to him and use them to cleanse him from negative energies. Then you fill him with positive energies.

The following illustration demonstrates a woman performing the *CCH* Light Technique on herself. She closes her eyes, envisions herself standing or lying, and pulls light energies to the envisioned body. The figure on the left is the woman herself and the one on the right is the energetic body that she envisions.

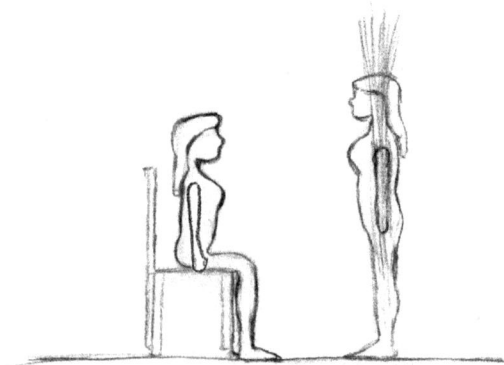

Illustration 3: A person who performs CCH Light Technique on herself

There are many ways in which *CCH Light Technique* can be performed. We will now practice "Light Shower."

CCH Light Technique: *"The Light Shower"*

This technique can be performed in a guided manner using the audio CD.

I ask that you sit up straight and close your eyes. Inhale through your nose and exhale through your mouth. Focus only on breathing.

When you inhale, the abdomen swells, and when you exhale, the abdomen flattens. Make sure that only the abdomen moves, swells, and flattens. The chest does not move.

Breathe in and breathe out five times.

Take a deep breath and exhale all at once. Relax your face; enable the skin of your face to rest, to fall, so there will be no expression on your face.

Relax your jaws, your tongue, and listen to your heartbeat. At the end of the exhalation, hold the breath for a second, listen to your heartbeat, and go on breathing.

Search for your heartbeat. Where do you feel it? Where do you hear it? Listen to your heartbeat from the inside.

Create complete silence and just listen to yourself from within.

Now, when you are connected and attentive to your inner self, *envision yourself* sitting up straight on the earth in an open space.

Inhale white light energy and exhale black energy. You only focus on breathing. Take in white energy and take out black energy.

A tube of light comes down from the heavens directly into your head. The tube enters through the head, passes through the center of your body, and continues into the earth. Those who look at you from the outside see a tube, rather than a person.

A waterfall of white light energy comes down from the heavens and into the tube. The waterfall is mighty and powerful. The light energy comes down through the tube and cleanses your body. It washes off all the negative energy or black energy.

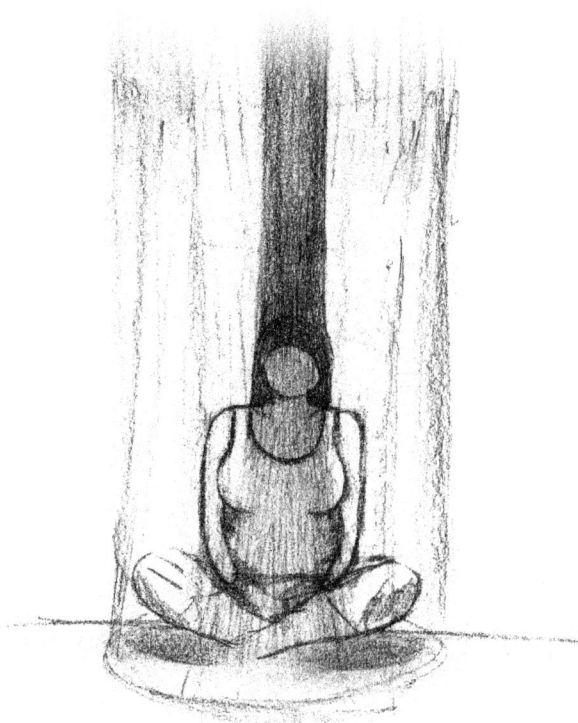

Illustration 4: Person connected to the earth and to the heavens through the tube of light

Perform "Light shower" every day. You may keep the waterfall of light with you throughout the day in order to fill yourself with positive energy. When you feel comfortable with this technique, you can perform it for your loved ones. As you saw yourself sitting in an open space, see the person for whom you perform the technique in the same way.

Summary

The divine spark is your center of life. Therefore, it is important that you treat it with respect and listen to its needs. You can treat it as a mentor who lives inside you and serves as your compass. It directs you to the best path for you. *Once the divine spark is in your everyday awareness, you will stop the race of life and think twice before doing things you are used to doing that might harm your divine spark. You can then choose to let go of your comfort and old habits in order to preserve the spark.*

When the divine spark's burning grows bigger, you will feel better, healthier, and more vital. You will contribute positively to yourself, to your loved ones, and to humanity.

When your divine spark burns, you are able to prevent suffering, stop the growth of existing suffering, and awaken your natural healing abilities. You have so much power in your hands to change and to influence. Therefore, it is so important that you focus on yourself; change and do whatever you can in your everyday life to preserve your divine spark.

In order for you to succeed in this task, I wish to remind you of several things that will help you maintain your internal burning, your divine spark. When you implement these things in your everyday life, you will wake up in the morning, and the thing that will motivate you will be the thought of your divine spark: how you can intensify it and what you need to do to increase the flame burning inside it.

- Every morning, when you wake up, close your eyes again and recall the existence of your soul and the divine spark that resides within it. Turn to your soul and ask it to unite with you. From this moment, keep the existence of the soul and the divine spark in your consciousness and act in ways that will serve them.

- Use the divine spark as much as you can. Be happy, create, help others, do things you love, and so on. Work with the card from the exercise "preserving the divine spark" on page 129.

- Invest in kindling the fire. In order to maintain and kindle the fire, you have to be constantly vigilant, perform work of personal growth, step out your comfort zone, and deal with the things that are difficult for you.

- Take responsibility for your thoughts, intentions, and actions, both towards yourself and towards others. The only one to bear the consequences is you, so do not look for others to blame for hurting your bonfire. Do not blame anyone for your suffering.

- Negativity towards yourself and towards your environment, from intentions and thoughts to actions, leads to the fading of your fire. Work with your cards from the exercise "Taking Out Negativity[4]," and "Preserving the Divine Spark.[5]"

- You can always move away from someone who gets close to your bonfire and tries to put it out. For example, if you do not feel good in someone's company, you do not have to remain his friend.

- Remember that the brighter your divine spark's burning, the bigger your children's divine spark's burning.

- Work with the energetic body and not against it, i.e., handle the cause of suffering and not only the symptom. You can also use one of the many holistic healing methods that can heal your suffering and help you work in the world of causes.

- Perform the "Light Shower" technique daily.

~~~

---

[4] See exercise "Taking out the negativity" on page 67.

[5] See exercise "Preserving the Divine Spark" on page 131.

Before we go on, stop and observe what you have received from this chapter through the following exercise:

Writing Exercise

Write in your notebook for five minutes:

- What did you learn in this chapter?
- What did you choose to do or to refrain from doing in your daily life?

If you have finished writing and you still have time left, close your eyes and ask yourself again: what did I get? What did I learn? What did I choose to do?

~~~

After completing the exercises in this chapter, you have advanced another step in being a healing parent. You understand the correlation between the burning intensity in the divine spark and the level of health of yourself and your loved ones. You also know what you can do or refrain from doing in order to keep the burning in your divine spark and to intensify it.

It is ideal for us to have the divine spark burn as it did on the day of our creation. In this state, we are healthy and use the power that lies within our spark for positive purposes of personal growth, creation, self-fulfillment, helping others, and more.

So what is the formula, what is the code that restores the divine spark as it was on the day of its creation? What do people need to do in order to remove all the "stones" that oppress their fire?

This is exactly what we are going to learn in the next chapter.

Part D

~

The Formula

Chapter 9

Restoring the Divine Spark

The great ball has given each of us a great gift, which is the divine spark. He has created us in a way that enables us to preserve it and make the most of it. You do not have to be a genius, wealthy, or have any special ability in order to keep the spark burning and make the most of it.

People live in the universe in different ways, according to their beliefs, their cultures, the home in which they were raised, their socioeconomic situation, their education, and their state of health. Despite all of these differences, we all have something in common, and that is the divine spark.

The great ball knew that in this world, each of his children would be provided with free will and each would create his own reality. In line with that, some things will benefit one person, while other things may benefit another. Yet with respect to the divine spark, *the great ball decided that there was going to be a fixed "formula" for preserving it, and whoever works with this "formula" will make the most of the spark and will earn physical, emotional, and mental health.*

The great ball wanted the one thing that affects human life the most and that embodies a great life force to be a simple element everyone could have.

This situation makes all of us equal. We all possess the divine spark and we all possess its potential. You must think that the formula for "preserving the divine spark" is complicated, exceptional, and innovative. I am happy to say that it is not! On the contrary; it is very simple and is found in everyone's grasp.

The formula for restoring the divine spark as it was on the day of its creation is:

Purity

Purity of the three bodies: the physical body, the mental body and the energetic body. I divide purity into three areas: purity of deeds, purity of thoughts, and energetic purity.

To illustrate the importance of the cleansing work you have to do in each body, I liken the person to a fruit tree.

The Energetic Body

In this body resides the soul; within it is hidden the divine spark.

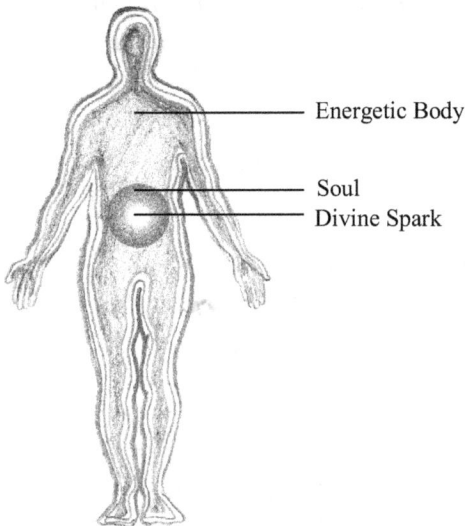

Illustration 5: the Energetic Body

I liken the soul of the human being to the seed of a tree.

The seed holds all the information of the tree that you want to grow. Such a tiny seed holds great power and influence over the tree that is about to grow. The healthier and stronger the seed, the stronger the roots it will sprout and the finer the fruit it will bear.

Therefore, the seed affects the roots and all the other parts of the tree.

Such is the power of your soul. Your soul holds all the information about who you are and your potential. The soul holds the power and influence over a person's life. *The purer the soul, the healthier and purer a person's actions and thoughts are, and the more the person can make the most of his divine potential.*

The cleansing work in the energetic body deals with the world of energies.

The purpose of cleansing the energetic body is to take out negative energies and thus protect the soul and use the soul's knowledge and potential.

A defective seed cannot use all of its potential. It may develop in a limited manner. The same holds true with us: if a person has in his soul energetic memories, the soul is not clean. He will therefore not be able to use all of his soul's potential. The cleaner the soul, the more the person is able to fulfill himself.

The Mental Body

The mental body contains the consciousness: thoughts, thinking patterns, conditioning: "if…then…"

I liken a person's thoughts to the tree's roots.

The roots affect the tree's life by nourishing the tree, thereby serving as its foundation. The roots funnel the "food" the tree needs in order to live. The stronger and healthier the tree's roots are, the more nourishment and the greater the foundation they can provide for the tree.

A person's thoughts are similar. A person's thoughts affect him by nourishing him and by becoming the foundation for everything he does. The more positive the thoughts, the more positively they nourish the person and the better and healthier the foundation they provide.

The cleansing work in the mental body deals with the world of thought.

The world of thoughts deals with two things: *positive thinking* and *focus*. By focus, I mean distraction-free thoughts. It is inconceivable that the tree's roots would be unfocused on their goal unless someone or something were to harm them. In this case, they would no longer be focused on nurturing the tree and will not able to bring benefit as they did.

A person's thoughts are similar: they must always be positive and focused on the person's goals so that he can achieve his heart's desires.

The Physical Body

The physical body contains the skeleton, all the body systems, body organs, tissues, body fluids, etc. This body also includes the feeling system.

Cleansing work of the physical body deals with the physical world.

I liken a person's actions to all the parts of the tree that are above ground. That is, the parts we can see. Actions are like the trunk, branches, leaves, flowers, fruit, and so on. Notice how many details there are in the physical world.

The healthier the seed and roots are, the healthier the entire tree is, and the more you can enjoy its fruit.

A person is similar. The more positive, healthy, and pure a person's intentions and thoughts are, the more moral, positive, pure, and good a person's actions are; the healthier and more harmonious a person's life is, the more he can make use of the Creator's abilities embodied in his divine spark.

~~~

Most of humanity is busy and preoccupied with the physical world, and thus most of humanity's energy is invested in that world.

It is important for a person to invest most of his efforts and time in the energetic world before he acts in the physical world. The energetic world is the world of seeds, the world of causes, the world of intentions. It is where everything begins.

A person who invests most of his energy in the energetic world will grow a big, healthy tree, full of fruits, in line with the healthy seed planted in the soil and the healthy roots created from the seed. Once the tree has grown and developed, all we have to do is cultivate it, protect it, and enjoy it.

Pay attention: The seed and roots are in the earth; not above ground, but within it, so no one sees them. This way there are fewer chances of someone sabotaging them. It gives them the chance to fully express their potential with no external interruption.

It is true regarding everything you create that involves intention and thought. Intention and thought conceal the greatest secret of your tree, the genetic code of your outcome, and therefore they need to be protected and not be exposed to all.

What do I mean? I recommend that you keep your thoughts and intentions from everyone but your nearest and dearest friends and family, such as your spouse. In business, I recommend that you involve only associates whose integrity you trust. I recommend that you not to let anyone penetrate your intent. It should only be found within you. What if a foreign element penetrates the roots of the tree? They will never be the same. They may be ruined immediately and the tree will not develop. That is exactly how you should treat your intentions and thoughts. Once you have let someone touch them, you have given permission for foreign energy to penetrate them. The result will no longer be in your hands alone.

Unlike the seed and roots, which are hidden and not exposed to others, all the other parts of the tree are exposed. Other people can and should touch them, be party to them and enjoy their fruit. When it comes to action, it is always right to share with other people. With the help of other people, you can boost the scope of your actions, enrich them, and develop them.

I will give you an example: several years ago, a pregnant woman who was carrying triplets came to me. Every single day she was exposed to horror stories about premature delivery, prolonged bed-rest, things that happened to other mothers and fetuses, and other intimidating stories and distractions. Everything she heard entered her and affected her health, and therefore the health of her fetuses.

I asked her to choose an intention that will serve her during the pregnancy. She chose to maintain her health and the health of her fetuses. I explained to her that the intention she had chosen was the seed she had planted. She should not let anyone harm it—this was her responsibility. She asked, "So, I can't speak about my pregnancy?" My answer was, "Of course you can." After all, she needed the help and support of anyone willing and able to provide it. However, she should not allow all the information that was out there to intrude on her seed.

I showed her that she was allowing all the intimidating details and horror stories that had nothing to do with her to enter her and create troublesome thoughts, such as, "What if I or the fetuses get hurt during the delivery?" "What will happen on their birthday?" and "How will we manage financially?"

I explained to her that all her worries had to do with future events, which were far from where she was, the pregnancy process. At this phase, her focus was to be on the pregnancy, so she could create the reality in the energetic world: keeping herself and the fetuses healthy. Dealing with anything else would sabotage the intention. This woman protected her seed and her roots the entire pregnancy and completed it keeping herself and her three fetuses safe and sound.

Dealing with the world of energies is also important in business. Business is not all about the physical world. Everything people do has intent, thought, and action. Also in business, the first thing you have to do is deal with intent. If you intend to start a business, ask yourself why you are starting it, what its goal is, what it may contribute to you, what it may contribute to others. The more you invest your time in the world of energies—the world of intentions—the more effortlessly your tree will grow and bear fruit.

To Summarize

The two worlds that preoccupy most of humanity are the physical world and the mental world. There is so much grime and chaos in these two worlds that we cannot see the existence of the energetic world, let alone deal with it and cleanse it. The primary purpose of our existence in this world is to use the knowledge and the potential of the soul and to contribute positively to the world. In order to succeed in this, we need to cleanse the soul. The soul helps us to cleanse, and it will do so in every possible way.

The playground for the majority of humanity is physical, and therefore the soul is also playing on that playground. It tries in every way to shout to the person, to direct him to change, to evolve and cleanse it, but most people are so preoccupied with their physical world that they are unavailable to hear the soul. To my regret, the soul is forced to shout louder and louder, and it does so through suffering.

Suffering is the means by which the soul brings the person face to face with the things he needs to cleanse. Suffering is something people cannot ignore. They feel the pain and understand they need to stop. They need to do something with themselves in order to remove suffering from their lives. When the person does not handle the source of suffering, the soul cries out harder so that the person sees what he needs to cleanse. As a result, many people get hurt. To my regret, among them are innocent and helpless children and babies.

My objective is to bring humanity back to play on the energetic playground, that is, to perform cleansing work of the energetic body. This leads to purification of the soul, to prevention of suffering, and to healing.

By working on the energetic body, people will prevent suffering in themselves and their loved ones, since the soul will no longer need to bring them face to face through suffering with what they need to cleanse. They will be attentive and will understand what they need to cleanse and correct in an easy and pleasant way; they will then be able to use the potential of their souls for positive causes.

Remember, the great ball created man in a way that enabled him to clean his thoughts, actions, intentions, and his energetic body every day, thus achieving purity and health.

Throughout the years, I have discovered the influence parents have on their children's lives.

I have discovered the connection between the children's physical, emotional, and mental suffering and their parents. And I have also found that when a parent goes through a cleansing and healing process, he prevents suffering in his children and cures their existing suffering. I have found that the formula that can release the children from suffering is their parent's purity.

The first step in being a healing parent is to take responsibility for your own purity, thereby affecting the health of your children.

The three bodies serve the person in his life and it is thus important to keep them pure. The three bodies affect each other; cleansing work on one body affects the other two.

In this book, we focus on cleansing the physical body and the mental body.

This cleanliness will give you direct access to the energetic body and will maintain its great vital force and keep it burning bright. The cleaner the mental and physical bodies are, the healthier they are. The energetic body does not need then to provide them with some of its fire for survival. The person can then use this power for personal growth, self-fulfillment, healing, helping others, and more.

So, how do we cleanse the physical body and the mental body? By using *Completion and Correction Healing (CCH)*[6].

CCH is an energetic way for healing, whose purpose is to prevent the suffering of people and to heal them. Through CCH, we perform work on the energetic body and influence also the physical body and the mental body.

The next two chapters are dedicated to cleansing the mental and the physical bodies. We will start with the mental body in the next chapter.

_____

[6] See "CCH Techniques" on page 130

Chapter 10

Cleansing the Mental Body

The mental body has great importance in a person's life. Anything a person performs involves a thought. The purer the mental body is, the more the person can control his thoughts, think positive thoughts, and focus on the things he does without his mind being distracted. When the mental body is cleansed, the person manages to concentrate considerable vital energy to achieve the reality he wishes to create in the physical world. Most of us have tremendous "noise" running through our minds. Most people do not notice what they think or what goes through their minds while they do things. As a result, they are controlled by thoughts. These thoughts manage their lives without them even noticing. A person who manages to control his thoughts controls his life and creates his reality.

The goal in cleansing the mental body is to be able to use the brain's capabilities in an empowering and positive way. To get the most out of the brain, you need to learn to quiet it and control it. I will now present to you ways to cleanse the mental body and achieve this goal.

Ways to Cleanse the Mental Body

We will learn three energetic ways to cleanse the mental body:

1. *CCH Light Technique*: "The Cone of Light"[7]

2. *CCH Technique*: Abolishing Negative Thoughts

3. *CCH Technique*: Extracting Negative Thoughts

A person who performs CCH Light Technique practices absolute control over his consciousness and unconditional giving. This way he develops inner listening abilities, inner vision abilities, accuracy, and concentration abilities.

CCH Light Technique: "The Cone of Light"

This technique can be performed in a guided manner using the audio CD.

Envision yourself lying on the warm earth in an open space. Breathe in white light energy and breathe out black energy. Each time you breathe out, envision yourself relaxing your body and let it lie comfortably on the earth. Focus only on breathing. When you breathe in your abdomen swells, and when you breathe out your abdomen flattens. Inhale white light energy and exhale black energy. You focus only on breathing. Take in white energy and take out black energy. The

---

[7] See "*CCH Light Technique*" on page 132

body takes on another dimension, much larger and wider.

See yourself pulling from the heavens a yellow ray of light and create around you a huge circle of yellow light energy. The circle of light is the size of two giant rooms, so compared to it, you are small. See yourself becoming larger and larger.

See yourself pulling from the heavens another yellow ray of light and connect it to the circle you are lying on, creating a huge cone of yellow light. Its base is on the earth, where you are lying down, and its tip is open to the higher worlds. If I ask you to spread your arms and touch the edges of the cone you cannot, because you are not big enough, so I ask you to see yourself becoming larger and larger.

From the heavens, pull a stream of white light energy. A great waterfall of white light comes down directly onto your abdomen. The light enters through the abdomen and spreads through the body. A tremendous amount of white light energy enters your body. The more light comes in, the more black energy gets out. Your body becomes bigger and wider. More and more white light energy enters your body, and your natural body contour diminishes.

At this stage, your body becomes larger. See yourself spreading your arms and touching the edges of the cone. Now you can, because you are huge. You can easily touch the edges of the cone with the tips of your fingers and toes.

I ask that you see yourself entering the cone of light and standing next to yourself. Now, see yourself entering your body. I want you to envision yourself walking inside your body as if it is a new street you want to familiarize yourself with. Wherever you go, the waterfall of light goes with you. If, for example, you are standing within your head, an immense amount of white light energy penetrates your head. You stay in your head until you feel the head no longer needs the light energy, and then you move on to the eyes, the nose, the throat, and so on. Your goal is to insert the waterfall of light into every organ in your body and envelop its exterior with light.

If a negative thought or a thought that is not connected to the healing work enters, I ask that you do the following: Envision yourself removing that thought from your head, wrap it in a bubble of white light energy, and throw it into the black hole. The black hole is a place in the heavens where all negative things go.

Remove anything you see inside the body, even if it seems lovely, and throw it into the black hole. You can pull a tube of light from the heavens and use it to draw out the thing you saw. If you see a person, take him out and perform a light shower on him.

Focus only on working with the light, enveloping every hair on your body with light, enveloping your skin with light. And again, if a negative thought or a thought that is not connected to the healing work enters, I ask that you envision yourself removing that thought from your head, wrapping it in a bubble of white light energy, and throwing it into the black hole. From this moment on, nothing negative can touch you.

When you finish performing this technique, leave yourself inside the cone of light, and remain in a state of awareness of the cone throughout the day. The cone will serve as protection from negative energy.

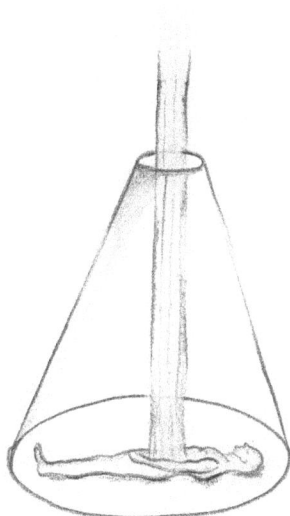

Illustration 6: Cone of Light

Perform the *CCH Light Technique* "Cone of Light" once a day for yourself. When you feel comfortable with this technique, you can perform it for your children. At this point, I do not recommend performing this technique on anyone other than your children.

CCH Technique: *Abolishing Negative Thoughts*

Thoughts have a direct impact on a person's life. Thoughts have the power to create reality and therefore negative thoughts have a negative effect on our lives.

The technique for abolishing negative thoughts we have studied (see page 69) allows you to remove such thoughts from your mind. If a negative thought enters while you perform *CCH Light Technique*, abolish it. If a thought enters that is not negative in and of itself but is still distracting or disturbing, envision yourself removing that thought from your head. Wrap it in a bubble of white light energy, throw it into the black hole, say to yourself *"I let go,"* and go on with your work.

This work helps significantly to clean your consciousness and helps you practice your ability to stay focused and concentrated on the things you do, without distractions. I thus recommend that you use this technique in your everyday life, while you cook, read a book, listen, walk, and so on. Get rid of bothering thoughts and inner conversations and focus on the things you do. In the beginning, you will feel you always get distracted by thoughts and find yourself "letting go," but after two weeks of daily practice, you will feel a change. You will feel there is more quietness and will be able to be more focused and concentrated.

CCH Technique: *Extracting Negative Thoughts*

This technique can be performed in a guided manner using the audio CD.

Every day, many thoughts go through your head. You are not even aware of most of them. These thoughts create "noise" and internal restlessness. The purpose of this technique is to release the congestion created in the mind, whether you are aware of it or not, and to create inner peace that will enable you to listen to yourself from within and to be relaxed and concentrated.

You can perform this technique on yourself as well as on your loved ones.

- Close your eyes and address your mental body: "Mental body, I ask that you bring up all the negative thoughts, all thinking patterns and all fears to the surface." Wait until you feel that everything has come to the surface. You may feel pressure in the head, eyes, ears, and so on, because a great amount of energy is building up.

- Envision yourself placing a big rectangular energetic magnet above your head.

- Address your mental body: "Mental body, I ask that you release everything you have brought up to the surface, all the negative thoughts, all the thinking patterns, all the fears, etc." Notice how the magnet magnetizes all the energy being released from the head. Energy may also be released from the ears and nose. When the magnet fills up with energy, it disappears and a new magnet takes its place. You can see the energy being released like black smoke or black bubbles. Wait for this process to end, until you feel or see that everything is out.

- Pull a waterfall of white light energy from the heavens and insert it into your head. Use it to perform a light shower, so if there is any negative energy or black energy in your head, it will come out.

- Bless yourself with good things.

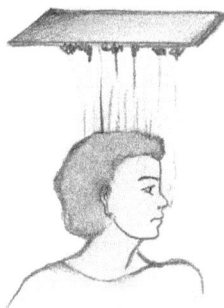

Illustration 7: Extracting Negative Thoughts

I recommend performing the technique every day.

You can teach your loved ones how to perform the technique for extracting negative thoughts themselves. You can also perform this technique for them.

Chapter 11

Cleansing the Physical Body

For the purpose of teaching, I liken people to tubes through which energy flows. The cleaner the tube, the more effortlessly the energy flows through it, and the more the person can use the energy for positive purposes such as personal growth, giving, listening, love, recuperation, and so on.

Whenever a certain issue is left untreated, it becomes an "object" that sits inside your tube, blocking the flow of energy. It can be any issue in any area of your life: things you wanted to say and never did, a letter you never sent, drawers you have not organized in a long time, or something you wanted to do but didn't.

Once you choose to deal with such an issue, you are taking the "object" out and making room for new energy to flow through the tube.

Anything that is not addressed in the physical world is a huge impediment for you, whether it has to do with relationships, delayed or unfinished tasks, or maintaining the physical body's health. A person who takes care of his relationships, handles his routine tasks, and cares for his physical body uses and directs his energies to fulfill his huge potential.

Suppose your desk has many unopened letters. You know you have to deal with these letters, but you are delaying the task. Your mind makes a note of the letters that need to be taken care of, and until you do, the thought about this task will not let go and plenty of energy you could have used for positive goals will be wasted.

When things are taken care of in the physical world, both the mental body and the energetic body are freed and the person can make the most of his potential.

Ways to Cleanse the Physical Body

I'll discuss three main parts in cleansing the physical body:

- Working on relationships
- Maintaining the physical body
- Addressing procrastination

Relationships

Relationships have a significant impact on a person's life. Cleansing relationships will relieve your heart and will allow you an open, free space for personal growth.

Communication is one of the most powerful ways to achieve personal healing and purification. There is communication above the surface—that is, words— and communication below the surface—that is, feelings and intentions.

People refrain from saying what is in their heart, they refrain from telling each other the truth, and they lie to themselves and to others by saying one thing and meaning another. People conceal what is in their heart while failing to understand that they are hurting themselves and those around them.

As long as a person says what he feels, and as long as there is a match between what he really feels and what he says, the other side feels comfortable and will accept the information given to him more readily.

The problems begin when a person does not say what is in his heart, or when there is a discrepancy between what he feels and what he says. Such situations lead to unease, misunderstandings, quarrels, power struggles, great frustration on both sides, and numerous other feelings and situations that could be avoided if people would only do one thing: speak the truth and say what is in their heart.

People avoid expressing how they feel for many reasons. They might fear that they will not be liked, or that they might hurt others. They might remain silent because they were taught to do so or because it is convenient.

We can improve, heal, fix, and cleanse so many things through communication. Your children are affected physically and emotionally from what you experience, even if you do not tell them a thing. It is therefore important that you assume responsibility for your life, observe your relationships with everyone who has influenced you throughout your life, and ask yourself one question: *Which conversation should I have?*

I wish to address your relationships with your parents, spouses, children, close friends, colleagues, and others.

Conversations can be held with the people living in this world and those living in the higher worlds, with people you are in daily contact or those with whom you are no longer in contact. The latter could be people to whom you wish to bid farewell or with whom you have a conversation you wanted to have but did not.

You may have been hurt by someone in the past or you may have hurt someone and you feel that you are not willing in any way to have a conversation with that person. Know that the conversations you find most difficult to engage in have the greatest potential in terms of cleansing your physical and your mental body. This cleansing will grant you immense internal freedom and will thereby lead to breakthroughs.

The next exercise will allow you to improve your relationships with others and to cleanse yourself through conversations.

Exercise: Relationships and Cleansing through Conversations

To perform this exercise, use the table on page 171.

1. Specify in the table the names of *all* your children as well as others close to you under the column "Person." Identify the types of conversations you need to have by checking the corresponding subject columns. The list of conversation topics is as follows: gratitude, forgiveness, farewell, clarification, request, frankness, confession, promise, sharing, and regret. For example:

   > Mother—a gratitude conversation and a regret conversation.

   > Father—a farewell conversation.

   Having no conversation marked means everything is so fine, there is nothing to talk about.

2. Write a letter to your parents and to an additional person with whom you have a conversation to perform. For example, write a letter of gratitude to your mother. Write what you are thanking her for. Another example can be a letter of farewell to a loved one from whom you separated when you were seventeen and did not tell him or her all that

was in your heart. Put on paper everything that is in your heart, everything you feel for him or her, and actually envision yourself saying goodbye.

3. If possible, call the people you mentioned or meet them and have the conversation in the physical world. If, for some reason, you cannot perform the conversation, close your eyes and have a telepathic conversation with them. Envision yourself having the conversation with them as if they were right beside you.

Person	Mother	Father	Spouse	Children				
Gratitude								
Forgiveness								
Farewell								
Clarification								
Request								
Frankness								
Confession								
Promise								
Sharing								
Regret								
No Conversation								

Table 1: Relationships

〰〰

If each day, you gave a new opportunity to yourself and to those you come in contact with, especially your loved ones, you would live in peace with yourself and those around you. Most people have prejudices towards others and these manage the relationship between them.

I want to perform with you a short observation and writing exercise that can help you cleanse the prejudices you have towards your loved ones, thereby opening a new page in your relationships. This will help you deal with your children and your spouse in an easy and positive way, thus maintaining domestic peace.

This exercise is called "Writing signs on the forehead." I will first provide some background.

Sign on the Forehead

A sign on the forehead is actually a label with which the child carries day after day, a label that affects his life. A parent—in his subconscious—imprints in the child's consciousness who the child is, and the child consequently often becomes such.

A negative label we put on our child is like a veil that prevents him from accessing his natural potential. For example, a parent decides in his subconscious that his child is cranky, and the child consequently becomes such. Each time the child steps out into the world, the first thing others see is the sign on his forehead, in this example, "cranky." Your goal is to become aware of these negative signs you may have placed on your children and replace them with positive signs that release them from the burden you put on them. This enables them to fulfill their natural potential.

In some cases, the label you placed from your subconscious on your children or your spouse empowers them, but in other cases, it does not serve them and even hurts them. At times, you will find that you put on the sign the exact thing you want to "change" in your child and by doing so you actually intensify this characteristic.

Now that you are aware of the influence you have on your loved ones by the signs you put on their foreheads, you can observe each of your children and your spouse and see what sign you put on their foreheads. If it is a negative sign, turn it to a positive one.

So, how do you change the sign? The following exercise will guide you in detail throughout the process.

Exercise: "Writing Signs on the Forehead"

1. Write in one column the names of your children and the name of your spouse.

2. Go over each of the names and check what sign you put on their forehead. Write next to each name whatever pops up.

   Start with the first child whose name you have written. Close your eyes and envision the child standing in front of you. There is no need for the child to be physically next to you.

   Ask yourself, "What sign did I put on the child's forehead?" Write in the notebook next to the child's name whatever popped up.

   Perform the same process on your other children as well as your spouse.

3. Change the sign according to need—if the sign does not serve the person, change it into a positive sign to serve him.

   If, for example, you put the sign "cranky" to your child, ask yourself "*what does he need to do or be in order not to be perceived by me as cranky?*" It might come up as "listening, calm, compromising, and more. Choose one thing. If you choose "listening," as far as you are concerned, when this child is "listening" he will no longer be cranky.

   Perform the same process on all the other family members.

4. Put a new sign on each person's forehead: envision him in front of you and envision yourself printing

on his forehead with gold colored letters what you chose as suitable for him. If you chose that your child is "listening," see the child in front of you. Print on his forehead "listening." Look at what you wrote, visualize the letters sinking into his forehead and create a seal of the word "listening."

Perform the same process on all the other family members.

By replacing the sign on a person's forehead, you can improve your relationship with him, make it easier on him, and enable him to be himself.

Reinforcing the Sign

I advise you to perform the exercise once every few months. To preserve the effect of the sign, every week envision yourself going over the sign on the forehead and reinforcing what you wrote, as if it faded or was erased.

～～

So far, I have shown how we can cleanse the physical body on the level of relationships. I will now present the second level of cleansing the physical body: maintaining it.

Maintaining the Physical Body

There are many aspects to maintaining the physical body. The four main factors are nutrition, hydration, sleep, and physical exercise.

1. Nutrition

Nutrition is one of the most powerful tools for maintaining proper human function. If you want to make a substantial change in your nutrition or learn more about nutrition, there are many books and professionals that can guide you.

Although plenty of knowledge is available about nutrition, I feel obligated to speak to you about the subject from a different point of view, which is *listening to the body's needs*.

I believe that every person can receive answers from within about the things that are right for him. For that reason, rather than going with a specific kind of diet, I tend to listen to my body and get answers as to what types of things are right for me.

Let us explore the subject of nutrition from several angles:

Consumption

One of the first things a person has to be aware of is what he consumes. Observe whether you consume things that you know are not healthy for you, like coffee, alcohol, cigarettes, drugs, or certain foods that may harm your health.

The following observation exercise will help you to do this:

✏️ Exercise: Observing Your Diet

1. Close your eyes and ask yourself: "What kinds of things do I put in my body that could harm my health?" Write everything that pops into your head.

2. Rank the items on your list according to their level of harm.

3. Circle three or more things you wish to work on. For each, see if you want to decrease its consumption or eliminate its usage.

Keep this list at hand. At the *moment of truth*, when you crave one of the items circled, ask your body several questions and wait for the answers:

- What do I need now?

- What am I missing in the physical body, the mental body, or the energetic body that makes me feel I need this particular thing?

- What must I fill myself with so I will not need this particular thing?

- What can replace the particular thing I crave?

Over-Eating

The majority of people eat more than their body needs. There are many reasons for that. Some people use food to calm internal restlessness, others eat in order to allay unpleasant feelings such as sadness, frustration, and boredom. To reduce the incidence of this phenomenon, ask your body two questions before you eat:

The first question is, *"Do I need to eat?"*

If the *answer is no*, ask your body, *"Body, what do you need?"* The answer can be anything—hydration, sleep, love, company, etc. If your body says you need company, close the refrigerator door and call a close friend.

If you get a positive answer, "Yes, I need food," ask a second question, *"Body, what food do you need?"* Before you eat what you *think* the body needs, make sure that your body really needs it. For example, if the answer is that the body needs something sweet, before reaching out for chocolate, ask your body if it needs chocolate. If the answer is "yes"—eat as much as you need. If the answer is "no"—ask your body what it needs instead of chocolate. It could be a teaspoon of honey or a date.

Foods that Would be Good to Avoid

I do not believe in complete bans, with the exception of things you are sensitive to or things that are toxic for you personally. However, there are several things I recommend using in moderation: sugar, alcohol, sweetened drinks, sodas, meat, dairy, yeast, and caffeine. If you choose to eliminate the things I mentioned, do it gradually. For example, if you are used to drinking three cups of coffee a day, reduce your consumption to two cups for the first week, and gradually eliminate it from your diet.

2. Hydration

Hydration is very important for maintaining the physical body. I recommend that you drink at least eight glasses of water a day.

3. Sleep

Sleep is extremely important to human health. It is important to maintain regular sleep habits. Allow the body to rest and prepare itself for the next day. While asleep, the body processes everything it has been through during the day. It is important to sleep at night, rather than during the day. Seven hours of sleep during the day are not as effective as seven hours of sleep at night.

Most adults need between six and eight hours of sleep a night, depending on the person's age.

4. Physical Activity

The fourth element that affects maintenance of the physical body is physical activity.

Physical activity is important for maintaining the various systems of the body, and also helps release energy trapped in the body. I recommend that twice a week you do aerobic exercise, such as walking, swimming, riding, or running. Once a week, do something that targets flexibility, such as yoga.

〜

When a person eats what he needs, in the quantity he needs, performs physical activity, drinks, and sleeps sufficiently, he preserves his life energy. He is healthier, more vital, and has enough energy to not only deal with survival but with things that contribute to himself and his environment.

So far, I have discussed two parts of cleansing the physical body; working on relationships and maintaining the physical body. I will now discuss the third part, which is addressing procrastination.

Addressing Procrastination

Most people put off to the next day chores, tasks, conversations, payments, and also their dreams. Things that are being put off pile up like layers of dirt in the physical world. These tasks may seem small and insignificant, and you might think they do not really need to be taken care of. It is important for me to tell you that these little tasks constitute a huge load that is burdening you and stopping you from fulfilling your potential.

I hear people say they do not have the power to perform simple tasks such as arrange the house, make themselves salad, go out for a walk, perform observation exercises, and more. Do you need so much power to perform these tasks?

If they ask their physical body, it will surely not agree with them. It has the power to make a salad, go for a walk, engage in a farewell conversation, and more. Moreover, the body will not understand why they do not perform what is good for them. Surely, this is not physical power, but an inner power within us. This power lies within the divine spark, and it has joy, hope, love, passion, and willpower. When these life forces are expressed in a person, he has the physical strength to do everything his heart desires[8].

So when we tend to postpone things, what do we need to do in order for the divine spark to burn?

Clean the physical body. Force yourself to continually act even if you lack the desire. Let go of

---

[8] See the summery of chapter "The Life Center of the Person" on page 140

any of your inner conversations that distract your mind from acting (see "Abolishing Negative Thoughts" on page 162). After two weeks of practice, you will feel something awakens in you, an inner strength that will give you energy to do things you have not done until now.

Exercise: Addressing Procrastination

Make a list of life areas, such as the following examples, and for each heading, note what you have to take care of:

- *Health*: medical tests.

- *Friendships and relationships*: invest in relationships, engage in conversations, go out, return calls, answer emails.

- *Children*: education, recreation, quality time.

- *Personal fulfillment*: hobbies, education, reading.

- *Sports*

- *Nutrition*

- *Housework*: tidy closets, drawers, kitchen, office, paperwork. Take everything you are not using out of the house and donate it to those who need it.

- *Donation*: donate money, volunteer, help others.

- *Repairs*: house or car.

- *Place of employment*: handle a crisis, report issues to management, change position, get a salary raise.

- *Finances*: banking, pension plan, savings, insurance, debts and loans, collection, and payments.

～

When a person lives in heightened awareness of his physical body and his mental body, when he listens to them and provides them with their needs in his daily life, these two bodies remain in balance and serve him throughout his life.

As long as the physical body and the mental body are healthy, the divine spark is free to act and make the most of the Creator's abilities inherent in it.

Epilogue
The Hourglass

Before we bid each other farewell, it is important for me to offer you a small gift—an hourglass. I am about to complete my guidance work for now and leave you to yourself, and therefore it is important for me to provide you with this modest gift, which will remind you of our way of life. Each one of you has your own hourglass. The hourglass will be there before you every day and remind you that time is passing. As long as the sand passes through it, you continue to live in this world and have the daily opportunity to correct and improve anything you choose. But you never know when the last grain of sand will drop. The moment the last grain touches the dune you created, time will end and you will no longer be living in this world. Yet then, amazingly enough, it will be possible to turn over the hourglass and start everything anew.

Each grain of sand that falls down is the present moment, yet it is also your future and your past, so that all times turn into one given moment which you live through.

Each grain of sand has meaning in your life and it serves the dune you are creating, so that the moment you turn over your hourglass and start everything anew, you will use each and every grain from your past and create a new dune.

The hourglass comprises a top part to remind you of the higher worlds located up above, and a lower part to remind you of this world. The sand that passes from the upper part to the lower part will also remind you of the connection between the higher worlds and our world, and of all the abundance and endless gifts that arrive in this world from the higher worlds.

The grains of sand are to remind you of the amazing light energies that come down from the higher worlds to our world; energies that empower, fill, and heal us.

The divine spark is the DNA of the great ball and it exists in every one of us. The strength of your divine spark depends only on one thing—your purity. The purer you are in your actions, thoughts, and intentions and the purer your energetic body and your soul, the more intensely your divine spark burns and serves you and your loved ones in a positive way.

In the cleansing process that you have started, you have taken great responsibility for your life, you have focused on yourself and have checked what you can improve and change in yourself so that your children will be healthier. In this process, you have enabled your divine spark to burn, and then magically you use it consciously day by day and you become happier, more patient, compassionate, loving, creative, peaceful, courageous, accepting, grateful, hopeful, and full of passion and energy.

Once the fog has cleared from your physical and mental body, you have created serenity within and around you and have realized that you are gifted. Now you are ready to get the next gift; an access to a new entrance door has been created. I invite you to take the next step in creating your reality by learning more of the *"Healing Parents"* knowledge.

I encourage you to go to the *Being a Healing Parent* website and find ways to learn more of the knowledge: www.healingparents.net.

All that is left for me to do now is to send you off with a blessing that you and your family will always live in peace and in complete health. I am delighted to have been given the privilege to impart the *"Healing Parents"* knowledge to the world; knowledge that shall lead humanity—through giant leaps—to physical, emotional, and mental freedom. Continue to live this way throughout your life and know that I am always with you.

With love,
Hannah

Index

About the Author

Hannah Pilnick was born and grew up in Israel. She is married and is a mother of three.

Hannah's discovery and development of the *Healing Parents* knowledge did not happen overnight. It is a lifelong path that is being paved and expanded with every passing day.

Hannah Pilnick graduated from college with a degree in homeopathy, and at the age of 25 began her life path of healing people as a classical homeopath.

At the age of 28, Hannah gave birth to her eldest son. From that moment on, she embarked on another journey, one that led her to discover who she was and to reveal her life's mission. As a new mother, Hannah took a yearlong vacation from her work as a homeopath and dedicated herself to raising her child. During this time, Hannah had the greatest discovery of her life. Through her son, she grasped the amazing connection between mothers and their children, and how parents influence the physical, mental, and emotional condition of their children. It was her love for her son and her strong desire to prevent his suffering that led her to discover that *the solution to children's suffering lies in their parents.*

From that point, Hannah went through a profound spiritual transformation that enabled her to realize that parents in general, and mothers in particular, can heal their own children. Through the documentation of thousands of cases Hannah healed, the idea kept taking shape. With the passage of time, Hannah understood that the concept of parents healing their own children is the most natural thing in the world. It was a concept that came from deep within her, awakening an awareness that had always been a part of her.

In 2008, Hannah Pilnick and her family moved to Los Angeles. Her husband Nadav left his career and joined her mission. Together, they have worked to make her dream of sharing this knowledge a reality. Over time, all of its many layers were revealed to her and became what is today known as the *Healing Parents* knowledge. The knowledge Hannah has accumulated over the years has been organized and presented to the world through her books and seminars.

Hannah continues to help parents mainly through seminars and books. Hannah and her husband Nadav have dedicated their lives to achieving the goal of preventing and uprooting suffering from the lives of all children by uniting people to work together to heal themselves and their loved ones.

Hannah Pilnick is currently working on the second book in this 3-part series. You can find out more about her work, lectures, and seminars on her website www.healingparents.net.

Book and Audio CD
Order Information

The Gift: The Power of Parenting (This Book)

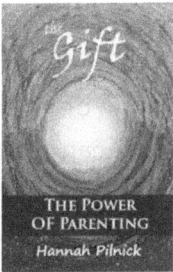

Format: *Paperback*

Go to
http://healingparents.net/clear/thegiftbook

or scan with your mobile:

Kindle version is available on Amazon.com

The Gift: The Power of Parenting | CCH Techniques

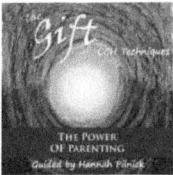

Format: *Audio CD*

Go to
http://healingparents.net/clear/thegiftcch

or scan with your mobile:

Learning More
Host a Live Seminar

Hannah Pilnick conducts numerous live seminars nationally and internationally year round.

To receive information about organizing a live seminar with Hannah, please complete the form below or go to www.healingparents.net/hostseminar. You can also

scan with your mobile ![QR code].

Your information

First Name: _____

Last Name: _____

Company: _____

Email: _____

Requested Seminar Information

Seminar City: _____

Preferred Date: _____

Alternate Dates: _____ _____

Email this form to info@healingparents.net
or **Fax** to (480) 247.5826

www.ingramcontent.com/pod-product-compliance
Lightning Source LLC
Chambersburg PA
CBHW051956090426
42741CB00008B/1411